QUALITATIVE AND MIXED METHODS IN PUBLIC HEALTH

QUALITATIVE AND MIXED METHODS IN PUBLIC HEALTH

DEBORAH K. PADGETT

New York University

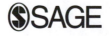

Los Angeles | London | New Delhi
Singapore | Washington DC

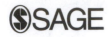

Los Angeles | London | New Delhi
Singapore | Washington DC

FOR INFORMATION:

SAGE Publications, Inc.
2455 Teller Road
Thousand Oaks, California 91320
E-mail: order@sagepub.com

SAGE Publications Ltd.
1 Oliver's Yard
55 City Road
London EC1Y 1SP
United Kingdom

SAGE Publications India Pvt. Ltd.
B 1/I 1 Mohan Cooperative Industrial Area
Mathura Road, New Delhi 110 044
India

SAGE Publications Asia-Pacific Pte. Ltd.
33 Pekin Street #02-01
Far East Square
Singapore 048763

Acquisitions Editor: Kassie Graves
Editorial Assistant: Courtney Munz
Production Editor: Astrid Virding
Copy Editor: Teresa Herlinger
Typesetter: C&M Digitals (P) Ltd.
Proofreader: Dennis W. Webb
Cover Designer: Bryan Fishman
Marketing Manager: Katie Winter
Permissions Editor: Adele Hutchinson

Copyright © 2012 by SAGE Publications, Inc.

Printed in the United States of America

Library of Congress Cataloging-in-Publication Data

Padgett, Deborah.

Qualitative and mixed methods in public health / Deborah K. Padgett.

p. cm.

Summary: "This text has a large emphasis on mixed methods, examples relating to health research, new exercises pertaining to health research, and an introduction on qualitative and mixed methods in public health. The book has an easy-to-read format and writing style and will also cover health focused research techniques, community participatory research, and will include boxed inserts pertaining to relevant real life examples"—Provided by publisher.

Includes bibliographical references and index.

ISBN 978-1-4129-9033-2 (pbk.)

1. Public health—Research—Methodology. 2. Social sciences—Research—Methodology. 3. Qualitative research. I. Title.

RA440.85.P335 2012
362.10973—dc23   2011019177

This book is printed on acid-free paper.

11 12 13 14 15 10 9 8 7 6 5 4 3 2 1

Contents

List of Table, Figures, and Boxes

Preface

Qualitative and mixed methods have never been more powerful or appreciated than they are today. This groundswell of interest has affected public health much as it has other professions, but with the unique twist that qualitative methods are making a comeback harking back to the early days of "shoe leather epidemiology." However, there has not been an accompanying increase in the availability of instructional texts targeted to the needs of public health students, practitioners, and researchers.

This book represents an attempt to fill the gap. An adapted version of an earlier text I authored entitled *Qualitative Methods in Social Work Research* (second edition, 2008, Sage), this text is devoted in its entirety to public health research. That said, many of its sections have been carried over from the earlier text. Qualitative and mixed methods have been adopted (and adapted) by many professions—education, nursing, medicine, social work, and psychology. What distinguishes these adaptations are the examples and applications specific to the profession's research agenda. Below are some examples of how this text reflects the current research agenda in public health.

What's New and Noteworthy in This Text

- A thorough-going revision by the author, who is an instructor and researcher in public health. This can be seen in the types of examples offered as well as the references and suggested readings.
- Expansive discussion of public health applications of qualitative and mixed methods such as community-based participatory research, photovoice techniques, and rapid assessment procedures
- An appreciation for the global interconnected nature of public health problems including an expanded treatment of cross-cultural and cross-language research

Continuities From the Earlier Text

- Conversational style
- Pragmatism rather than ideology with regard to "what works"
- Emphasis on observation as well as interviewing
- Emphasis on the importance of strategies for rigor in qualitative methods
- Detailed description of six of the most commonly used qualitative methods (ethnography, grounded theory, case studies, narrative analysis, phenomenological analysis, and community-based participatory research)
- Inclusion of specific illustrative examples from my own funded research on breast cancer and homelessness
- A broad, multidisciplinary perspective that draws on the social and behavioral sciences as well as diverse health professions
- Emphasis on the specifics of coding and thematic development
- Discussion of qualitative data analysis (QDA) software types and how this software can be used
- Detailed guidelines on writing a qualitative or mixed methods research proposal in the Appendix
- Exercises at the end of every chapter that can be done either individually or in a classroom setting
- Recommended readings and web-based resources for additional learning

Background to This Text

This book reflects yet another step in a personal journey. My doctorate in anthropology, postdoctoral training in public health, and federally funded qualitative and mixed methods research on breast cancer and homelessness all came together to make this text possible. But what made this text inevitable (at least in my estimation) was a basic need I had as an instructor in the Masters Program in Global Public Health here at New York University (NYU). Begun in 2004, the program has prospered and I have had the privilege of teaching two of its core courses: Global Issues in Socio-Behavioral Health and Qualitative/Field Methods in Public Health. It was the latter course that led me to pursue writing a text by revising a book I had previously authored for social work researchers.

Involvement in NYU's global public health program has given me license to redevelop and reinvigorate my anthropological and public health knowledge by teaching students from a variety of backgrounds, both professional and national. In any given class, I encounter students from up to 15 different nations, many of whom are physicians and few of whom have had exposure to social science theories and qualitative methods.

Meanwhile, qualitative methods have become increasingly visible in the scientific journals and conference programs of the professions—education, nursing, social work, public health, medicine, occupational therapy, and so on. These methods have also become a multidisciplinary meeting ground for researchers in the social sciences, humanities, and other professions who eschew the singular dominance of quantification in favor of more naturalistic approaches.

While the public health research literature began to reflect this transformation in the 1990s, public health curricula have been slower to register the change. Courses in qualitative and field methods have become more common, but are frequently the result of individual faculty interest rather than systematic inclusion as a linchpin of the curriculum.

In the case of my own public health program, the need for a required course in qualitative methods arose not only from my self-interested advocacy but from the program's emphasis on capstone experiences in the field, far from the controlled conditions of a laboratory or experiment. For students embarking upon projects in a village in India, a maternity hospital in Ghana, or an inner-city part of Brooklyn, the need for cultural competence and methodological feasibility rendered most quantitative studies either not possible or not appropriate. Developing countries (as well as poverty-stricken regions of Western countries) rarely have the resources to gather health systems data (much less keep it "clean and ready" for researchers to use). Put another way, the gap between sophisticated health informatics systems characteristic of some (but not all) Western nations and the realities of public health research "on the ground" is enormous, and it is consequential.

Public health students embarking upon field projects armed solely with knowledge of randomized clinical trials and the latest statistical modeling techniques regularly confront this reality. Moreover, mounting a household or other survey of sufficient sample size for statistical analyses requires extensive resources and local acceptance (neither of which is easy to obtain these days). Even those fortunate enough to have access to health systems data frequently find it unsatisfying to sit in an office working with the data, removed from the lively and unpredictable interactions that make being in the field come alive.

Successful capstone projects in our program have consistently relied on focus groups, observation, and in-depth interviews with key informants and local community members. The ease of entry and the rapport afforded by qualitative methods—matched with limited time and resources—have made their utility readily apparent. But their payoff is also substantive, not simply a matter of expedience.

What Is Distinct About This Book

What does this text offer beyond what is already available? The rapid increase in public health initiatives funded by governmental sources such as the U.S. Agency for International Development has led to the publication of field guides online (DeMarco, Carswell, Hornowski, & Snider, 2005; Mack, Woodsong, MacQueen, Guest, & Namey, 2005). There is also a hard-copy field guide available (Ulin, Robinson, & Tolley, 2005). The text you are holding is, to my knowledge, the first to provide academically oriented instruction in qualitative and mixed methods in public health. By this I mean the content portrays these methods in a broader and deeper context—their social science origins, their theoretical and epistemological linkages, and their varied types and uses in public health. Field guides play an essential role in providing the basics, but academic instruction in public health is best served by comprehensive coverage of qualitative methods and their disciplinary ties to public health theories and concepts. This "bringing the outside in" perspective is where the influence of the social and behavioral sciences in public health enters the picture. Acquiring skills in using these methods remains a key aim of this book, but it is also designed to address the broader educational needs of students and new learners.

Recent events in the world—wars, popular uprisings, and epidemics—have brought home the need for research that is relevant to human experience. Public health researchers who want to make a difference have plenty of work to do. Broad-based aggregate data and quantitative analyses are needed to address population-level (large sample) problems. But grassroots perspectives from (and involvement with) those most deeply affected are also essential to understanding and acting to resolve these problems. Qualitative and mixed methods contribute in vital ways to making this happen.

Scope and Organization of the Book

As the reader will see in Chapter 1 and beyond, the term *qualitative methods* covers a wide variety of techniques and approaches. These diverse approaches coexist as a loosely connected family—a bit contentious at times, but always interesting and capable of making a significant contribution.

The chapters are roughly organized around the sequential steps involved in carrying out a qualitative study—even though the reader is cautioned that qualitative inquiry is rarely if ever a linear or predictable process. Chapter 1 gives a brief history of the theoretical and disciplinary origins of qualitative methods (in general as well as specific to public health). It also grounds the reader in epistemological and other sources of diversity within qualitative methods and sets the stage for what follows. Chapter 2 includes a description of six of the most commonly used qualitative approaches (ethnography, case studies, grounded theory, narrative, phenomenological, and community-based participatory research) to give the reader an overview of options from which to choose. Chapter 3 introduces the reader to mixed methods, or the incorporation of both quantitative and qualitative methods within the same study. Chapters 4 through 8 take the reader through the various stages of carrying out qualitative research: study design and sampling (Chapter 4), ethical issues (Chapter 5), entering the field and conducting observation (Chapter 6), interviewing and use of documents (Chapter 7), and data analysis and interpretation (Chapter 8). Chapter 9 is devoted to rigor in qualitative research, and Chapter 10 provides guidelines for writing up the study and disseminating its findings. Finally, the Appendix presents the basics of writing a qualitative or mixed methods proposal based on my experiences and the experiences of others.

A Few Words on Writing Style and Terminology

This Preface seems the best place to make a few points about writing style and use of terminology. First, I have tried to incorporate sensitivity to gender, ethnic, and other forms of diversity throughout the text. Second, the awkwardness of nonsexist usage has led me to alternate use of masculine and feminine pronouns and to use plural pronouns on other occasions. Finally, I have a strong preference for the term "study participant" with occasional substitutions of "respondent" or "interviewee," depending on the context of the discussion. The researcher is also a "study participant," so this choice is not perfect but it seems most suited to the interactive dimension of qualitative research.

The reader has probably already noted my liberal use of the first person. This more informal style of expression has become commonplace in qualitative research and is a natural consequence of the trend toward greater self-disclosure and transparency. After years of being confined by the restrictive writing of quantitative reports, I am pleased to be able to write more informally and playfully. By the same token, I have tried to avoid unnecessary jargon and have highlighted key terms with italics to underscore what is important.

Although comprehensive and inclusive of the diversity present in qualitative methods, this is still an introductory text designed to complement specialized works, classroom instruction, and hands-on experience. I have included examples as well as exercises throughout to aid the reader seeking more in-depth understanding of (and experiences with) specific approaches and techniques.

One overarching goal of this book is to promote greater methodological transparency as well as rigor. Paying attention to what happens during a qualitative study—and meticulously documenting decisions and procedures even and especially when they change—ensures that others can understand how the findings were produced. There will always be an element of "trust me" in qualitative inquiry (compared to "trust the methods" in quantitative studies) due to its reliance on the researcher-as-instrument. But it is incumbent on qualitative researchers to minimize this tendency and demystify their methods as much as possible. This book is intended to help move us farther along in that direction.

When all is said and done, textbooks and coursework are necessary but never sufficient—mastery in qualitative and mixed methods requires real-world experience. With this in mind, I invite you on a journey of discovery that I hope will keep you engaged and informed.

The Audience for This Book

This book has its origins in the growing enthusiasm for qualitative and mixed methods in public health. While oriented to public health students and professionals, the chapters take an ecumenical approach and can be useful to a variety of practitioners and researchers in related fields including medicine, nursing, dentistry, and allied health professions. Intended for graduate students, faculty, and other professional researchers, this book provides a solid foundation for carrying out rigorous and relevant research.

Acknowledgments

The many students and colleagues I have encountered as a professor in social work and public health have provided me with ideas and encouragement for which I am deeply grateful. Among them, Upal Basuroy, Lalitha Ramanathapuram, and Laura O'Hara stand out. I offer my gratitude to the research team and study participants of the New York Services Study, the former including Andrew Davis, Ana Stefancic, Courtney Abrams, and Ben Henwood. The study, funded by the National Institute of Mental Health (#R01 MH69865), provided many of the examples used herein. Finally, I sincerely appreciate Kassie Graves at Sage Publications and the reviewers listed below whose comments and suggestions made this book possible.

Rosemary M. Caron, *University of New Hampshire—Durham*

Sally J. Guttmacher, *New York University—New York*

Stephanie B. Jilcott, *East Carolina University—Greenville*

Jay Maddock, *University of Hawaii-Manoa—Honolulu*

Michael Reece, *Indiana University-Bloomington—Bloomington*

Mark Swanson, *University of Kentucky—Lexington*

1

Introduction

The field of public health has never been as widely known or popular as in recent years. On a global scale, the spread of HIV/AIDS beginning in the 1980s gave public health enormous impetus and visibility. Much like infectious diseases from earlier eras, HIV/AIDS was deeply enmeshed in environmental and behavioral contexts. If left unaddressed, the disease promised to engulf large portions of the world's population.

Yet today's most enduring and pervasive public health problems are far more mundane, e.g., poor sanitation and water quality, malnutrition, and the everyday violence of grinding poverty. The 20th-century reign of the germ theory of disease etiology, with its emphasis on curing over prevention and laboratories over communities, has been tempered by these realities and by the vast increase in chronic diseases such as hypertension, diabetes, and cancer. Similarly, the dominance of quantification, in which ever-more sophisticated measures and statistics are expected to capture the full range of human experience, has given way to a more nuanced and thoughtful matching of methods with the problem at hand as well as with the people and places experiencing it (Baum, 1996; Rapkin & Trickett, 2005).

Enter Qualitative Methods

A colleague once astutely remarked that virtually anyone can read and appreciate qualitative research—its narrative reporting style makes it appear easy to carry out. By comparison, a quantitative study relies on complicated

1

statistical analyses that require prior knowledge to decode their meaning. Yet the appealing end product of a qualitative study represents the culmination of intense involvement and intellectual labor. Whether used alone or in a mixed methods study, qualitative methods have become central to research in public health. This, in a nutshell, is what this book is all about.

The term *qualitative methods* is a relative latecomer to the methodological lexicon, coming long after ethnography and other forms of naturalistic inquiry had been on the scene. There is no "one size fits all" qualitative method to make the definitional task easier; the aphorism "a mile wide and an inch deep" (quantitative) versus "a mile deep and an inch wide" (qualitative) is useful heuristically if a bit simplistic.

Nowadays, qualitative research can be referred to as a family of methods in which some members are more compatible than others. Some members have been around for a long time (e.g., ethnography, case studies, and grounded theory). Others such as narrative analysis, constructivism, and phenomenological approaches are newer on the scene.

And what about *mixed methods?* Rising appreciation of qualitative methods has made them attractive to researchers seeking to use both quantitative and qualitative approaches to maximize their understanding of a phenomenon. Now considered a separate form of inquiry with its own experts and terminology (Creswell, 2007; Pope, Mays, & Popay, 2007; Tashakkori & Teddlie, 2010), mixed methods research has followed closely on the heels of the popularity of qualitative methods.

Differences From and Similarities to Quantitative Methods

To varying degrees, qualitative methods entail assumptions and approaches that set them apart from quantitative research. At the risk of oversimplifying, the distinctions are as follows:

- Insider rather than outsider perspectives
- Person-centered rather than variable-centered
- Holistic rather than particularistic
- Contextual rather than decontextual
- Depth rather than breadth

Qualitative methods emphasize being inductive over being deductive. They favor naturalistic observation and interviewing over the decontextualizing approaches of quantitative research. As such, they imply a degree of closeness and an absence of controlled conditions that stand in contrast to the distance and control of traditional scientific studies. Qualitative research is predicated on an "open systems" assumption where the observational context (and the observer) is part of the study itself (Manicas & Secord, 1982). In contrast, quantitative research favors a closed (or controlled) system approach in which every effort is made to neutralize the effects of the observational context (including the observer).

Qualitative studies seek to represent the complex worlds of respondents in a holistic, on-the-ground manner. They emphasize subjective meanings and question the existence of a single objective reality. Furthermore, they assume a dynamic reality, a state of flux that can only be captured via intensive engagement. A qualitative report is a *bricolage*, a pieced-together, tightly woven whole greater than the sum of its parts.

Doing qualitative research requires an unparalleled degree of immersion by the researcher as the instrument of data collection. Unlike the pre-coded, standardized questionnaire, the qualitative researcher must be a sensitive instrument of observation, capable of flexibility and on-the-spot decision making about following promising leads.

Drawing these contrasts between quantitative and qualitative methods is a necessary heuristic device to highlight what makes qualitative methods unique. There are also similarities between the two; some believe that the differences are more stylistic than epistemological (Flaherty, 2002, p. 513). Among their shared characteristics, both quantitative and qualitative approaches are empirical, relying heavily on firsthand observation and data collection to guide findings and conclusions. Second, both are systematic. Contrary to some misperceptions, qualitative research is not haphazard or unfocused, nor is it prescriptive or predictable. This dynamic tension between flexibility and serendipity on the one hand and methodological rigor on the other makes qualitative research exciting and challenging. Qualitative studies start out as inductive but need not remain exclusively so; such studies often alternate between induction and deduction (Morgan, 2007).

Paradigmatic "Camps" in Qualitative Methods

As qualitative inquiry has flourished, so have its internal divisions. The intellectual fermentation that resulted can be reasonably (and somewhat simplistically) described as producing three paradigmatic "camps": post-positivism, constructivism, and critical perspectives. In this section, we review how, when, and why these three camps arose.

Positivist reasoning and quantification—the drivers behind the explosion of scientific and technological inventions in the 20th century—came under withering criticism from academic thinkers in the latter part of that century. Concerns about the assumptions of value-free objectivity and a verifiable reality gave rise to a "post-positivist" stance acknowledging the presence of values (admittedly as sources of bias), the provisional nature of knowledge, and the influence of the "knower" on what is known. Although more commonly adopted by social scientists rather than the "hard sciences," the term *post-positivism* and what it represents are, largely by default, the epistemological backdrop to scientific inquiry over the past four decades.

The broad-based critique of logical positivism drew adherents from 20th-century philosophy (particularly phenomenology) but owes most of its impetus to the post-1960s upheaval among French intellectuals including Jacques Derrida, Michel Foucault, and Jean Baudrillard. A number of philosophers and social scientists in Europe and the United States joined a burgeoning postmodern movement (Harding, 1987; Rabinow & Sullivan, 1979). In anthropology, Geertz (1973, 1988) and Clifford and Marcus (1986) inspired a profound reexamination of ethnography in light of previous assumptions of "naïve realism." In sociology, Berger and Luckmann's treatise on *The Social Construction of Reality* (1967) provided a revelatory counterpoint to positivism. Last but by no means least, Lincoln and Guba's landmark book *Naturalistic Inquiry* (1985) and their subsequent collaborations with Norman Denzin set definitional boundaries around "qualitative methods" as separate from and largely in opposition to positivism and quantitative methods. Invoking Kuhn's (1970) observations on paradigm shifts, these proponents argued that epistemology was paramount and positivism was incommensurable with the nascent approach of constructivism. By the late 1980s, disciplinary boundaries were becoming blurred as social scientists embraced the humanities—philosophy, literature, and the arts—and produced works such as poetry, dance, and autobiography.

By the 1980s, learning about qualitative methods meant being drawn into paradigm arguments in which one was urged to declare one's allegiance, with the most prominent voices calling for a rejection of post-positivism (Denzin & Lincoln, 1994). For these opponents of post-positivism, the label given to their resistance—postmodern, anti-foundational, post-structural, constructivist, interpretivist—mattered less than the message being promulgated. *Constructivism*—a belief that human phenomena are socially constructed rather than objectively "real"—proved to be a liberating force for many researchers (Charmaz, 2006; Denzin & Lincoln, 2005). It has led to reexamination and reflexive critiques of what is meant by "race," "gender," "deviance," and "mental illness" among many other social "facts." Exposing the ways that such concepts are invented and reified has been a prime source of new understanding in the social sciences. The rub comes from taking this point of view to mean that there is no reality attached to concepts such as "race" or "gender." Although few would argue that "race" is one of humanity's most troubling inventions, it has an objective existence manifested in the discriminatory treatment of individuals with darker skin common to so many societies. Similarly, "poverty" has multiple meanings—absolute and relative—and all have consequences for health and well-being (Link & Phelan, 1995).

The third epistemological camp is explicitly devoted to research on inequalities as an ideological and moral imperative. Critical approaches such as feminist, Marxist, race, and queer theories (Harding, 1987; Ladson-Billings, 2000; Madison, 2005; Olesen, 2000) are united in their commitment to the disempowered. *Critical theorists* point to inequalities based on gender, race, social class, and sexual orientation as hidden (and not-so-hidden) subtexts of much of the knowledge produced by Western science. Left unchallenged, these inequalities are reinforced through power differentials that are virtually self-perpetuating.

By implication or by deliberate intent, postmodern critiques embraced qualitative methods as the "answer" to the flaws and reductionism of positivist research, and the constructivist and critical theory camps became aligned with the postmodern movement (although some individual members kept their distance). Their hortatory language and indictment of all things positivist set the stage for the rise of *pragmatism* (more about this in the following section).

This discussion of paradigmatic camps would be incomplete without a concluding observation: Paradigm debates are far more evident in books and articles *about* qualitative methods or *about* the dominance of Western science than in research reports *featuring* these methods. Put another way, situating one's methodology within a certain epistemology is a choice that many researchers do not make (or at least do not make explicit). This has been a source of chagrin for paradigm purists but less a concern for paradigm pragmatists (whether self-declared or by default). Meanwhile, quantitative researchers have manifested little interest in joining the debates, perceiving little need to justify or question the dominant assumptions under which they operate.

The Pragmatic Middle Ground

It is possible to appreciate aspects of postmodernist critiques (especially those focused on the privileges of power) without endorsing the whole paradigmatic package. After all, doubts about quantification and traditional research designs have emerged from within the positivist camp (D. Campbell, 1979) as well as from without (Abbott, 1997).

Several qualitative researchers (H. Becker, 1996; Creswell, 2007; Patton, 2002; Tashakkori & Teddlie, 2010) have gone on record favoring pragmatic philosophy as a less ideological middle ground. A uniquely American phenomenon developed by John Dewey, Charles Peirce, and Jane Addams (among others), pragmatism in its nascent form was a reaction to metaphysical arguments on the nature of Truth and Reality (Cherryholmes, 1992; Menand, 2001; Rorty, 1998; West, 1989). Rather than take a stand on such philosophical conundrums, pragmatists accept the fallibility of knowledge development, elevating utility over ideology or philosophy. Thus, one can be comfortable with the notion that there are occasions when reality claims can and should be made ("genocide in Rwanda"), when a presumed reality practically cries out to be deconstructed ("deviant behavior"), and when multiple subjective meanings can produce a broader understanding of something ("post-traumatic suffering"). Put another way, all concepts are human inventions, but some are more socially contrived and consequential than others.

Anthropologist Nancy Scheper-Hughes (1996) argued in favor of a "strong scientific and moral imperative to get it right" (p. 891). Thus, "while reality is always more complex, contradictory and elusive than our limited theories and methods can possibly encompass, some things remain incontestably *'factual'*" (p. 891). Scheper-Hughes goes on to discuss the need to boldly report acts of genocide and violence that beset many of the world's poor and displaced.

Research Methods in Public Health: The Rise of (and Return to) Qualitative Approaches

The Place of Research in Public Health Education and Practice

Research in public health draws heavily upon its core discipline of epidemiology and the scientific method, but it was not always thus. Early studies were more likely to use "shoe leather epidemiology" and field observation than large-scale surveys and surveillance efforts. A convergence of events in the 20th century produced what came to be the norm in public health research methods. First was the development of statistical analyses and operationalism, or measurement. When paired with experimental designs and large-scale surveys, the uses and benefits of quantification were readily apparent. Second, the emergence of lifesaving antibiotics, vaccines, and surgical procedures inspired confidence in randomized controlled trials as never before. Medical advances and space age technology lent credibility to science as having a seemingly infinite capacity to explore and explain. Finally, the growth of a public health infrastructure made record keeping on morbidity and mortality—the core data sources of biostatistics—routine governmental activities. The U.S. Centers for Disease Control and Prevention (CDC) began in 1942 to monitor malaria control and take over many of the activities previously carried out by the Rockefeller Foundation. At times overshadowing the effects of basic improvements in sanitation and nutrition, the medical model approach to inquiry, i.e., clinical trials and statistical analyses, came to dominate public health research. Recently, however, the pendulum has begun to swing back toward public health's origins in more naturalistic investigations (Faltermeier, 1997).

Box 1.1 **Public Health Practice and Research: Making the Distinction**

Public health entails practice and research—and the boundaries between the two are not always clear. In 1999, the CDC issued guidelines for distinguishing research from non-research in public health (www.cdc.gov). Acknowledging that the usual descriptors of "systematic" or "data collection and analysis" do not serve the purpose, the CDC guidelines point to intent as pivotal, i.e., the *intent* to generate or contribute to generalizable knowledge. Citing three public health activities—surveillance, emergency response, evaluation—the guidelines note that these may involve systematically collecting and analyzing data that at some point become generalizable. But these activities do not cross the threshold of being research unless they go beyond helping the patients or population being served.

To illustrate how difficult it is to make the distinction, look below at a recent listserv ad for a public health internship with a "rapid program quality assessment"

(Continued)

(Continued)

conducted by a world relief organization working in Africa. The intern's responsibilities, spread over an 8- to 12-week period, include the following:

- Help develop training package for data collectors (1 week)
- Participate in data collection and field supervision (1–2 weeks on-site)
- Perform data entry and cleaning (1 week on-site)
- Carry out data analysis (2 weeks)
- Draft a report documenting assessment findings (1 week)

The intern would be expected to assess the knowledge and skills of community
health workers (CHWs) as well as the quality of supervision of the CHWs by their
affiliated health centers. Skills being sought include familiarity with software
(e.g., STATA, MS Outlook, and Excel) and writing, editing, and researching skills.

Commentary: This description appears to be all about research. However, according to CDC guidelines, it is not because the findings are directed solely to improving services within the organization; i.e., they constitute public health practice.
Note the short time frame involved. Such a quick turnaround presents a standing
challenge to researchers' traditional need for sufficient time to mount a credible
project and carry it through to completion. This is, however, common in public
health programs, especially those carried out in developing countries.

The "New Epidemiology": Multiple Causations and Multiple Methods

The turn to more flexible methods has run parallel to a paradigm shift in
epidemiology that rejects "the myopic focus of biomedicine on micro-
level causes of diseases in individuals (e.g., human genes, infectious
agents)" (Inhorn & Whittle, 2001, p. 554). Critics charge that mainstream epidemiology and its associated methods ignore larger eco-social
contexts (Krieger, 2001). If health problems are viewed as due to individual
responsibility, then health solutions will be sought through changing
unhealthy beliefs and behaviors. Larger structural inequalities—gender,
race, socioeconomic—escape notice as lying outside the realm of existing
etiological frameworks. The example of tobacco use illustrates this quite
well. As noted by Baum (1996), establishing the link between smoking and
lung cancer required traditional quasi-experimental designs well-known

to epidemiologists, but well beyond this important etiological break-through are the psychological, social, and cultural factors influencing the decision to smoke (or not). At the same time, individual decisions about smoking occur within larger influential contexts—it would be myopic to ignore the powerful effects of billion-dollar advertising campaigns by tobacco companies.

Also escaping notice in the rush to quantification were the sensitive, subjective, and biographical details of individual lives that lend a deeper and more nuanced understanding (Faltermeier, 1997). Standardized measures are weak approximations when it comes to capturing the suffering of a cancer patient, the thrill of smoking crack cocaine, or the deep trauma of rape. To ignore all things that cannot be measured is to leave public health bereft of aspects of the human experience underlying the onset and course of diseases, addictions, and traumas.

The limitations of quantitative methods are also apparent when a study is focused upon complex, dynamic, and changeable phenomena. Notwith-standing efforts to examine multilevel systems (Nastasi & Hitchcock, 2009; Trickett, 2009) using nested variables and hierarchical modeling (Raudenbush & Bryk, 2002), the vast majority of studies use individuals as units of analysis and cross-sectional or static designs. A constraint related to longitudinal studies arises from the inaccuracies of recall in retrospective designs and high rates of attrition in prospective designs. Finally, there are the challenges of statistically modeling repeated observations over time.

On balance, both quantitative and qualitative methods have something to offer. Surveys supply much-needed aggregate information on individuals, households, neighborhoods, organizations, and entire nations. Yet they fall short in assessing individuals as they live and work *within* their households, neighborhoods, organizations, and nations.

Box 1.2	An Enduring Public Health Parable: The River Story

A widely invoked parable of unknown origins but told well by Irving Zola (quoted by John McKinlay, 1986) is the "River Story." The storyteller relates a harrowing tale of saving a drowning man in a rushing river and dragging him to shore, only to see a struggling woman in the water followed by others in

(Continued)

(Continued)

similar dire straits. Repeated dives into the cold river to save the growing number of victims leaves the storyteller exhausted with no time to go upstream to see why so many people are falling into the river in the first place. Or perhaps to see why so many are being pushed into the river? And what about those who managed to swim to safety on their own?

The lasting power of this metaphor for public health lies in its illustration of misplaced priorities and the need for primary prevention. The story illustrates the importance of structural (upstream) factors such as inequalities that place individuals in harm's way in the first place. Of course, one could counterargue that individuals imperil themselves through bad habits and unhealthy life-styles; i.e., they recklessly venture into the river assuming it will not engulf them later downstream. Just discussing this parable and its possible iterations—along with the distinction between upstream and downstream—offers a valuable "teaching moment" in public health.

Proponents of the "new epidemiologies" were drawn from the ranks of community health and AIDS activists as well as feminists and others who pointed to the pernicious effects of "structural violence" (Castro & Farmer, 2005; Inhorn & Whittle, 2001; Leung, Yen, & Minkler, 2004). *Structural violence* refers to historical and socioeconomic forces that place certain individuals at greater risk of health and other problems and make them less likely to receive treatment. Their vulnerability may be due to racism, sexism, poverty, sexual orientation, or some combination of these. That social conditions such as poverty can be a "fundamental cause" of disease and premature mortality (Link & Phelan, 1995) is a direct refutation of etiologies dependent on individual culpability, whether genetic or behavioral.

Although this newer approach might seem to be neutral with regard to methods, this is far from the case. As noted by Inhorn and Whittle (2001),

the "opening" of epidemiology requires that epidemiologists join forces with anthropologists, sociologists, historians, and feminist scholars, who are not only more theoretically oriented but who also value alternate, qualitative forms of data (e.g., illness narratives, life histories, participant observations, structured observations of doctor–patient interactions, popular media accounts, historical documents) that give context and meaning to epidemiologists' more quantitative analyses. (p. 558)

This alignment of critical perspectives, social science theories, and qualitative methods is an indication of shared values and resistance to the notion that clinical trials and statistics were all that was needed for the public health researcher's toolkit. As we will see in this book, qualitative researchers in public health and in general may or may not subscribe to critical perspectives. Indeed, the family of qualitative methods is diverse and its adherents are independent-minded when it comes to paradigm allegiance.

Evidence-Based Practice in Public Health: The Role of Qualitative Methods

Evidence-based practice (EBP) has become a powerful movement sweeping through health care (Ericsson, 2000). Rooted in biomedicine, EBP challenges the practicing professions to offer evidence-based interventions and abandon those found to be ineffective or harmful. Determinations of effectiveness are made using a hierarchy of evidence that places randomized controlled trials (RCTs) at the top. Public health has joined the EBP movement, as have many health professions (Waters & Doyle, 2002).

With the rise of EBP, meta-analyses and systematic reviews have gained favor as a means of synthesizing extant research. The Cochrane and Campbell Collaborations (the former dedicated to health and the latter to social welfare, education, and criminal justice) have generated numerous reports from such syntheses showing the effectiveness (or lack thereof) of interventions ranging from breast cancer screening to antipsychotic medications (see www.cochrane.org and www.campbellcollaboration.org).

Public health practitioners often work in settings where RCTs are difficult or impossible to carry out (Victora, Habicht, & Bryce, 2004; Waters & Doyle, 2002). Perhaps not surprisingly, many have joined other health professionals in questioning whether RCTs can provide definitive answers to "what works" given the complexities of health problems and their solutions (Victora et al., 2004). Overarching concerns about EBP center on the narrowness implied by scientific definitions of "evidence" and the methods deemed adequate for its determination. In particular, the devaluation of "indigenous ways of knowing" is considered a hindrance to working with communities to reduce health disparities (Cochran et al., 2008). From a qualitative research standpoint, the elevation of experimental evidence from "gold standard" to "only standard" is worrisome because it leaves little or no room for the depth and flexibility of qualitative studies (Morse, 2006). Although proponents of EBP have expressed interest in accommodating qualitative methods, progress has been slow and understandably hobbled by the distinctive nature of qualitative studies.

The EBP movement clearly has its limitations, although its underlying premise is difficult to repudiate. Who, if anyone, would want to use a surgeon who ignores the latest research findings and prefers to rely solely on personal experience? In retrospect, empirical research on Bruno Bettelheim's "cold mother" explanation for autism might have prevented the damage it caused to parents and families of autistic children.

At the same time, acceptance of what EBP has to offer need not lead to dismissing other forms of knowledge, including subjective meanings, cultural beliefs, and discursive revelations (Cochran et al, 2008). A step in the right direction has been taken by some leading quantitative researchers who have gone on record favoring qualitative methods as a "touchstone of reality" in community-based interventions (Hohmann & Shear, 2002, p. 205). The survival and relevance of the EBP movement depends on fostering appreciation for multiple methods.

Theoretical and Conceptual Frameworks in Qualitative Inquiry

Some Are a Better Fit Than Others

The relationship between qualitative research and theory is complex and subject to varied opinions (Anfara & Mertz, 2006). On the one hand, allowing one or more theories to drive the inquiry deprives a study of what qualitative methods do best—explore the unknown or find new ways of understanding what is known. On the other hand, qualitative studies do not take place in a conceptual vacuum.

It is helpful to distinguish among several versions of what is meant by "theory" in public health. This variety in meaning is due to differing degrees of explanatory ambition, conceptual abstraction, and openness to multiple interpretations. These differing meanings include (1) grand theories having a sweeping scope and high level of abstraction (e.g., Freudian or Marxist theory); (2) mid-range theories used in research on behavioral and organizational change (e.g., Bandura's social learning theory or Rogers' diffusion of innovation theory); (3) conceptual frameworks that offer organizing principles and evocative concepts, without being strongly predictive (e.g., the health belief model and the Andersen and Newman model of service utilization); (4) critical theories (feminist, race, queer, etc.) that address societal inequalities; (5) theories that operate as an "open system" and are not deterministic (e.g., Blumer's symbolic interaction theory or Bronfenbrenner's social ecology theory); and (6) inductively derived mid-range theories that have been the foundation of grounded theory methodology (Glaser & Strauss, 1967).

Perhaps not surprisingly, versions 1, 2, and 3 are least suited for qualitative studies to the extent that they are determining rather than orienting in their intent and use. Psychological and biomedical theories present a distinct challenge because they are focused on identifying and solving specific problems of an intrapsychic or physical nature. As mentioned earlier, critical theories (version 4) have been adopted by many qualitative researchers but are less about methodology than ideology. In contrast, versions 5 and 6 are a closer fit for qualitative research given their openness to inductive reasoning. Version 6 is only possible with qualitative research.

Concepts do not have to be enmeshed in theoretical frameworks to be useful, e.g., *stigma, identity,* and *social support.* There are few concepts more widely used (and misunderstood) in public health parlance than *social capital.* Popularized by Putnam in his book "Bowling Alone" (2000), social capital has been put forth as a multidimensional concept representing the tangible benefits of social relationships. The notion that social capital is central to explaining variation in health and mental health has been both embraced and decried, but its staying power is undeniable (Szreter & Woolcock, 2004).

As Barney Glaser (2002) aptly noted, such staying power and the capacity for representation and evocation make a concept transcend localized description. Morse (2004) goes further to note that concepts fulfill a number of vital functions, enabling the researcher to engage in pattern recognition, synthesis, constant comparison, and generalization. Ultimately, concepts comprise theories, fitting together like the pieces of a jigsaw puzzle (Morse, 2004). Their contribution to a qualitative study is never guaranteed, but without conceptual frameworks coming before (and most importantly, from) data analysis, the study's contribution is severely diminished.

Theoretical Thinking in Public Health Research: The Role of the Social and Behavioral Sciences

Though traditionally closely allied with medicine, public health has increasingly drawn on the social and behavioral sciences to understand complex public health problems (Willis et al., 2007). Leading theoretical frameworks from these disciplines—critical theories, ecological theories, behavioral theories, organizational theories—have found their way into public health research and served as a bridge between the conceptual worlds of health and psychosocial concerns (Willis et al., 2007). For example, psychological theories have shaped behavioral health interventions targeting tobacco use, substance abuse, and obesity.

Attention to psychological, social, and cultural factors offers a far more comprehensive (and complicated) portrait of public health problems beyond the basic mechanisms of biology. The AIDS epidemic in the 1980s opened the door to recognizing *syndemics*, or co-occurring health problems rooted in larger structural forces (Singer & Clair, 2003). Support for the notion of a syndemic comes from convergent evidence showing that health problems are more heavily concentrated among the poor and marginalized, whether due to biological diseases, toxic environments, violent injuries, mental illness, or substance abuse. In this context, attributions of "risky lifestyles" (unsafe sex, substance abuse, overeating, etc.) are contextualized as involving more than individual choice. Qualitative methods have been central to these multifactorial conceptions of public health problems.

The Place and Timing of Theories in Qualitative Studies

In further contemplating the role of theories in qualitative studies, a few questions arise:

- What (if any) theoretical ideas and concepts are to be used?
- When do they inform the study?
- How are they incorporated into the study?

Answering these questions can depend on the study's epistemological foundation as well as its approach and methodology. Figure 1.1 depicts this flow from the abstract to the concrete, with examples given for each phase indicated by Roman numerals. It is fair to say that many qualitative studies start at Phase IV and bypass the earlier three phases altogether.

Figure 1.1   The Foundations and Processes of a Qualitative Study

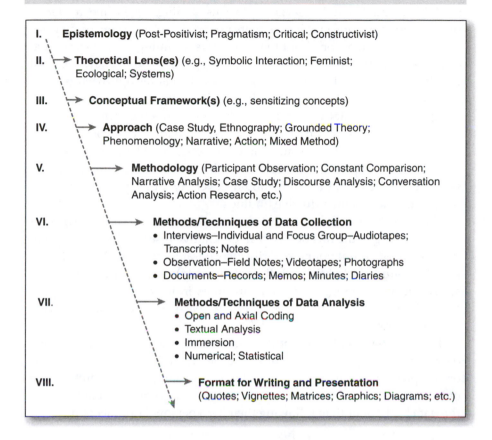

I.   **Epistemology** (Post-Positivist; Pragmatism; Critical; Constructivist)

II.   **Theoretical Lens(es)** (e.g., Symbolic Interaction; Feminist; Ecological; Systems)

III.   **Conceptual Framework(s)** (e.g., sensitizing concepts)

IV.   **Approach** (Case Study, Ethnography; Grounded Theory; Phenomenology; Narrative; Action; Mixed Method)

V.   **Methodology** (Participant Observation; Constant Comparison; Narrative Analysis; Case Study; Discourse Analysis; Conversation Analysis; Action Research, etc.)

VI.   **Methods/Techniques of Data Collection**
- Interviews–Individual and Focus Group–Audiotapes; Transcripts; Notes
- Observation–Field Notes; Videotapes; Photographs
- Documents–Records; Memos; Minutes; Diaries

VII.   **Methods/Techniques of Data Analysis**
- Open and Axial Coding
- Textual Analysis
- Immersion
- Numerical; Statistical

VIII.   **Format for Writing and Presentation** (Quotes; Vignettes; Matrices; Graphics; Diagrams; etc.)

The "what" question builds on this discussion with the additional point that qualitative researchers may simultaneously draw on several theoretical frameworks and concepts as "lenses" through which the study's data and ideas are refracted. This is a good reason for adopting a multidisciplinary perspective because an openness to ideas from a variety of sources lends freshness and creativity to a qualitative study. However, it also entails making decisions and taking risks.

How might this work? A study of family caregivers of Alzheimer's patients might draw on concepts from social exchange theory (such as reciprocity), from the research literature (such as coping, burden, and stigma), and from the researcher's own orientation (such as resilience). These represent a place to start but hopefully not to finish, their survival dependent on whether they earn their way into the findings (Charmaz, 2006). The study's potential is fully realized when its findings invite the reader to understand caregiving in a deeper, more nuanced, and even surprising way.

The "when" question about theories refers to timing (i.e., whether theories influence the study from the beginning or are held in abeyance until the data analysis and interpretation phase). The latter approach is often used in phenomenological research, which favors immersion and fresh insights. Most qualitative approaches, however, involve some theoretical ideas and concepts early on in the process; these ideas and concepts may remain during the analyses and some new ones may be incorporated as well. In a sense, Phase II in Figure 1.1 can be seen as cascading down over subsequent phases, although it should never lay a heavy hand or crowd out serendipitous and inductive findings.

The "how" question is the most challenging (and least discussed) question pertaining to the role of theory in qualitative research. As a rule, theories are imported but not necessarily incorporated into qualitative studies (i.e., they are held lightly and discarded easily). In the early stages of a study, theories provide leads and directions in formulating study questions. There are few guidelines to follow; each researcher must decide how much (or how little) to do this.

The importation of theoretical ideas becomes more complicated in the data analysis stage because by this time, emergent ideas begin to support or supplant previous concepts and ideas. Qualitative researchers are obliged to be careful when making the "how" decision (i.e., going where the data lead rather than following their own personal predilections).

Reasons for Doing Qualitative Research

What kinds of research interests are best suited for qualitative research? There are several scenarios possible. These are not mutually exclusive, nor are they exhaustive, but they do provide some of the more common arguments for using qualitative methods.

1. You are exploring a topic about which little is known—especially from the "inside" perspective. This approach is the hallmark of qualitative methods.

There are many fascinating research topics (e.g., risky sex among men "on the down low" who proclaim themselves heterosexual, women who are impregnated by rape and decide to keep the child, parents who adopt disabled children from developing countries, family members who participate in assisted suicide). Such topics need not be pristinely untouched. What is important is that too little is known about them and an in-depth understanding is sought.

2. You are pursuing a topic of sensitivity and emotional depth. Public health professionals routinely encounter human crises and dilemmas that require empathy and understanding. These professional experiences provide a wellspring of ideas for research where the use of a standardized, numerical rating would be inappropriate or insensitive (Morse, 2010).

For researchers interested in behaviors considered taboo or stigmatized, qualitative methods may be the only plausible approach. Ethnographic studies of heroin dealers, gang members, and sex workers portray the lives of individuals who are not likely to cooperate with the usual forms of survey research. Moreover, studies of sensitive topics need not be confined to the fringes of polite society—one can "study up" as well as "study down" (e.g., community leaders after a natural disaster, or doctors who abuse prescription drugs). Of course, members of an elite population are often the hardest to study, capable of using their power to limit access in ways that the poor cannot (Hertz & Imber, 1995).

3. You wish to capture the "lived experience" from the perspectives of those who live it and create meaning from it. When researchers seek *verstehen* (deep understanding), they pursue studies that are *emic* (i.e., focused on the insider point of view, rather than *etic* [the outsider's perspective]). Examples include studies of the lives of older homeless women, the experiences of chronic pain patients, or the dangers surrounding military nurses working in a war zone

4. You wish to get inside the "black box" of practice, programs, and interventions. Perhaps not surprisingly given the push for accountability in health care services, program evaluations have become heavily focused on quantitative outcomes. Yet qualitative methods have a secure place in evaluation research (Padgett, 2009b). They are a natural fit with formative evaluation given their capacity to identify unforeseen effects of a new program that may hamper (or pave the way to) its implementation. Likewise,

qualitative methods in process evaluation shed light on how (not whether) a program succeeds or fails.

So much of professional practice plays out in messy, unbounded ways that do not lend themselves to preformed standardized measurement. The deeply communicative aspects of practitioner–client relationships are fertile ground for narrative analysis, the daily hubbub of an emergency room practically cries out for ethnographic observation (C. Hall & White, 2005), and the successful pairing of program theory and staffing can set the stage for a case study of best practices. Qualitative studies do not yield "hard" outcomes, but their naturalism and agility can produce a description that emerges organically from the practice setting.

5. You are a quantitative researcher who has reached an impasse in explaining or understanding. It is striking how often unanswered questions emerge during quantitative studies that call for qualitative research. My earlier quantitative research on ethnic differences in mental health services help-seeking frequently led me to fall back on a "cultural" explanation calling for more in-depth examinations of how members of ethnic groups perceive mental illness and the service delivery system (Padgett, Patrick, Burns, & Schlesinger, 1994). The insurance claims database we accessed was of no use for such a purpose.

6. You are seeking to merge advocacy with research. *Action* and *participatory research* are devoted to countering the effects of oppression and social injustice (Fals-Borda & Rahman, 1991; Freire, 1973; Reason & Bradbury, 2007); the recent popularity of community-based participatory research (CBPR) in public health is an example of the continued relevance of activist approaches dating to the 1970s (Leung et al., 2004). Although the nature of the researcher–community partnership varies considerably, an overall goal is to use research methods on behalf of social change. Both qualitative and quantitative methods can be used, but the central premises of action research are closely aligned to the relationships common to qualitative research.

In summary, there are many sound reasons to do qualitative research— some or all of the aforementioned scenarios may underlie a particular study. There are also reasons *not* to pursue qualitative research. Foremost among these is that the topic of interest may be better served by quantitative designs such as experiments or surveys. Second, anyone seeking qualitative methods as "the easy way" should be forewarned—the intensive labor and immersion required are reason enough to think twice.

Desirable Qualities and Skills in the Qualitative Researcher-as-Instrument

The qualitative researcher's unique position as the instrument of data collection imposes special burdens as well as opportunities.

Indeed, a qualitative study's success depends heavily on the researcher's personal qualities as well as intellectual capacity. The absence of structure allows wide latitude—to reach creative heights as well as the depths of intellectual paralysis or disturbing biases. A few qualities that an individual can have or cultivate make the conduct of qualitative research more successful. These include flexibility; self-reflection (reflexivity); and an ability to multitask in an iterative, nonlinear way.

Flexibility is a state of mind and of behavior (Ely, Anzul, Friedman, Garner, & Steinmetz, 1991) well-suited to the unpredictable, ever-changing landscape of naturalistic inquiry. Respondents may suddenly refuse to cooperate with an interview, put off being interviewed, or not show up at all. They may divulge shocking information, make sexual overtures, or suddenly turn the questioning around to put the interviewer on the spot. Data analysis may (and often does) lead to new directions and new study participants. One's favorite ideas or theories may not be borne out and, as a result, may have to be cast aside. The strength and success of qualitative research lie in the researcher's ability to go with the flow rather than always try to control it.

Reflexivity, the ability to critically examine one's self, is a central preoccupation in qualitative research. As noted by Michael Agar (1980), "the problem is not whether the ethnographer is biased; the problem is what kinds of biases exist and how can their operation be documented" (p. 42). Examining one's biases requires ongoing vigilance throughout the course of the study.

Finally, a qualitative study is guaranteed to produce vast amounts of raw data awaiting management and analysis from its earliest stages. The *ability to multitask* on a number of levels (i.e., to simultaneously collect and analyze data, keep track of what is happening via memos, and remain open to new insights and the bigger picture) must be present and constantly nurtured in the researcher-as-instrument.

In addition to personal capabilities, certain skills are essential to the qualitative research enterprise. Among these are the skills of observation and interpersonal communication. Both of these are common elements of a practitioner's training, but their application in qualitative research follows a different track. When teaching qualitative methods to public health students, I ask them to carry out an exercise in participant observation. They must go to the public place of their choice (a park, subway station, street fair, playground, etc.), observe the action for one hour, and write up field notes describing what they have seen. What a departure this is for them! Trained to focus on problem resolution, they must be passive observers and not intervene. The open-ended nature of qualitative observation can be awkward and even painful for individuals who are more comfortable with the "filters" of clinical training and the authority to guide what happens.

The interpersonal skills of empathy and sensitivity, important in public health practice, are put to somewhat different ends in qualitative research. Rather than foster engagement for treatment or health promotion purposes, these skills enable listening as part of the pursuit of knowledge and understanding. This requires a degree of humility and subordination of self that takes some getting used to.

Finally, two of the most essential skills needed in qualitative research are the interrelated abilities to think conceptually and write well. The need to think abstractly and create new perspectives is the sine qua non of qualitative methods. Termed *theoretical sensitivity* by Glaser (1978), this refers to the ability to give interpretive meaning to data, to separate the wheat from the chaff.

Formulating ideas and developing concepts and theories depend on the ability to write. Experienced qualitative researchers often remark that the act of writing (i.e., recording memos and writing up preliminary ideas) is central to the success of a study. A well-developed sense of humor helps enormously in qualitative research, particularly the ability to laugh at oneself. One's vulnerability and inexperience when entering the field almost guarantee that there will be mistakes; some of them will be funny in the eyes of others. (Anthropologists invariably have stories of abject humiliation and jokes made at their expense.)

Finally, there is the capacity for collaboration. With the exception of doctoral dissertations, the days of the lone investigator are fading fast. Although individuals can and still do carry out qualitative studies with little outside assistance, the scope and sophistication of research make teamwork and collaboration increasingly the norm. Interdisciplinary participation is especially welcome in a qualitative study in which the richness of insight is enhanced by differing perspectives.

Introducing the New York Services Study (NYSS): A Qualitative Study of Homeless Mentally Ill Adults in New York City

Being fortunate enough to receive a 4-year, all-qualitative grant from the National Institute of Mental Health (NIMH) in 2004 was, for me, the culmination of long-standing personal and professional interests. A postdoctoral-funded professional retooling at Columbia University's School of Public Health in the mid-1980s provided training in quantitative methods and opportunities to collaborate with senior researchers analyzing data from a survey of New York City's homeless shelters at the height of the homelessness crisis. Serendipitously, a fellow researcher, psychologist Sam Tsemberis, decided to return to clinical work and conduct homeless outreach for a public hospital in New York City. This position ultimately led Dr. Tsemberis to start the first-ever "Housing First" program for the homeless mentally ill in 1992.

This new program, Pathways to Housing, Inc., became part of a federally funded randomized trial that compared the Pathways model to the dominant "continuum" approach (in which the homeless mentally ill must become clean and sober and live in congregate care with accompanying rules and requirements). The New York Housing Study examined housing stability and other quantitative outcomes across the comparison groups from 1997 to 2001. As it happened, few meaningful group differences were found at the study's end beyond that of greater housing stability for the Pathways subjects. This raised questions about the impact of Housing First, but also about whether the quantitative measures were capturing what was really happening. (Anecdotal reports by the study's interviewers and interviewees pointed to greater dissatisfaction and life problems among the control group participants who remained either in congregate care or on the streets.)

Intrigued by this discrepancy, I drew on my previous quantitative research on homelessness and my self-proclaimed expertise in qualitative methodology to prepare an all-qualitative R01 grant proposal for submission to the National Institute of Mental Health. Success in obtaining funding took a revised submission that ultimately garnered positive reviews.

The New York Services Study (NYSS) began in September 2004 with staff consisting of a full-time project director, three interviewers, and two part-time transcribers. The NYSS had three specific aims that revolved around identifying what worked and did not work in the service delivery system intended for homeless persons with serious mental illness and co-occurring substance abuse. Specific examples from the NYSS will be used throughout this book to illustrate various facets of a qualitative study.

Summary and Concluding Thoughts

Beginning with a rich historic background synonymous with ethnography (and, later, grounded theory), qualitative methods grew ever more diverse and multidisciplinary. Beginning in the 1970s, the various non-quantitative methods that became known collectively as "qualitative" came into full flower—with phenomenological and narrative approaches joining ethnography, grounded theory, and case studies. Soon thereafter, mixed (quantitative-qualitative) methods brought the possibility of synergy and multiple perspectives.

As with other professions, public health has becoming more open to and appreciative of qualitative and mixed methods. Coinciding with this change has been a "paradigm shift" that has transformed public health as it has become more attuned to global problems and the social, economic, and cultural dimensions to these problems. This more expansive vision of health and well-being, coupled with a concern for "ground up" perspectives, opens the way to more broadly conceived and inclusive approaches to public health research. There is a parallel here. Just as qualitative methods have their roots in (and derive nourishment from) the social sciences, public health has witnessed a resurgence of social science influence. The methodological balance still tilts heavily toward quantitative methods (in the social sciences as well as in public health), but there is increasing attention to more naturalistic field methods attuned to the myriad ways that health problems are manifested and ameliorated.

This chapter introduced key topics that cut across the landscape of qualitative inquiry, including the role of theories and concepts, reasons for using qualitative methods in public health, and capabilities and skills that enhance one's ability to succeed as a qualitative researcher. Addressing each of these orients the reader to the complex and discretionary aspects of qualitative methods—all of which will be in evidence in the chapters to come.

EXERCISES

In the classroom, break into small work groups. (This can also be done individually.) Choose a research topic of interest in public health and discuss the following:

1. The various epistemological positions or "camps" described in this chapter. How might your topic be framed in terms of these paradigms (post-positivist, constructivist, critical)?

2. What advantages do qualitative methods bring to the study? (Hint: Refer to the reasons for doing qualitative research in this chapter.)

3. What theories or concepts discussed in this chapter might be applicable to the topic?

4. What qualities and skills do members of the group possess that will help them engage in a qualitative study?

Additional Readings

Becker, H. (1998). *Tricks of the trade: How to think about your research while you're doing it.* Chicago: University of Chicago Press.

Bodgan, R., & Taylor, S. J. (1998). *Introduction to qualitative research methods* (3rd ed.). New York: Wiley.

Bourgeault, I., Dingwall, R., & de Vries, R. (Eds.). (2010). *The SAGE handbook of qualitative methods in health research.* Thousand Oaks, CA: Sage.

Corbin, J., & Strauss, A. L. (2008). *Basics of qualitative research* (3rd ed.). Thousand Oaks, CA: Sage.

Crabtree, B. F., & Miller, W. L. (1999). *Doing qualitative research* (2nd ed.). Thousand Oaks, CA: Sage.

Creswell, J. W. (2007). *Qualitative inquiry and research design* (2nd ed.). Thousand Oaks, CA: Sage.

Creswell, J. W., & Plano Clark, V. (2010). *Designing and conducting mixed methods research* (2nd ed.). Thousand Oaks, CA: Sage.

Denzin, N. K., & Lincoln, Y. S. (Eds.). (2005). *The SAGE handbook of qualitative research* (3rd ed.). Thousand Oaks, CA: Sage.

Emerson, R. (2001). *Contemporary field research: Perspectives and formulations.* Long Grove, IL: Waveland Press.

Flick, U., & Salomon, A. (2010). *An introduction to qualitative research* (4th ed.). London: Sage.

Flick, U., von Kardorff, E., & Steinke, I. (Eds.). (2004). *A companion to qualitative research.* London: Sage.

Green, J., & Thorogood, N. (2004). *Qualitative methods for health research.* Thousand Oaks, CA: Sage.

Hesse-Biber, S., & Leavy, P. (2010). *The practice of qualitative research* (2nd ed.). Thousand Oaks, CA: Sage.

Huberman, A. M., & Miles, M. B. (Eds.). (2002). *The qualitative researcher's companion.* Thousand Oaks, CA: Sage.

Israel, B. A., Eng, E., Schulz, A., & Parker, E. A. (Eds.). (2005). *Methods in community-based participatory research for health.* San Francisco: Jossey-Bass.

Liamputtong, P., & Izzy, D. (2005). *Qualitative research methods* (2nd ed.). London: Oxford University Press.

Mack, N., Woodsong, C., McQueen, K. M., Guest, G., & Namey, E. (2005). *Qualitative research methods: A data collector's field guide.* Research Triangle Park, NC: Family Health International. Available at http://www.fhi.org/en/rh/pubs/booksreports/qrm_datacoll.htm

Marshall, C., & Rossman, G. B. (2011). *Designing qualitative research* (5th ed.). Thousand Oaks, CA: Sage.

Merriam, S. (2002). *Qualitative research in practice: Examples for discussion and analysis.* New York: Wiley.

Miles, M. B., & Huberman, A. M. (1994). *Qualitative data analysis* (2nd ed.). Thousand Oaks, CA: Sage.

Minkler, M., & Wallerstein, N. (2008). *Community-based participatory research for health: From process to outcomes* (2nd ed.). San Francisco: Jossey-Bass.

Morse, J. M. (Ed.). (1994). *Critical issues in qualitative research methods.* Thousand Oaks, CA: Sage.

Padgett, D. K. (Ed.). (2004). *The qualitative research experience.* Belmont, CA: Thomson.

Patton, M. Q. (2002). *Qualitative research and evaluation methods* (3rd ed.). Thousand Oaks, CA: Sage.

Rossman, G. B., & Rallis, S. F. (2003). *Learning in the field* (2nd ed.). Thousand Oaks, CA: Sage.

Schwandt, T. (2007). *The SAGE dictionary of qualitative inquiry.* Thousand Oaks, CA: Sage.

Seale, C., Gobo, G., Gubrium, J. F., & Silverman, D. (Eds.). (2004). *Qualitative research practice.* London: Sage.

Silverman, D. (2010). *Doing qualitative research* (3rd ed.). London: Sage.

Stringer, E. T. (2007). *Action research* (3rd ed.). Thousand Oaks, CA: Sage.

Tashakkori, A., & Teddlie, C. B. (Eds.). (2010). *SAGE handbook of mixed methods in social and behavioral research* (2nd ed.). Thousand Oaks, CA: Sage.

Tolman, D. L., & Brydon-Miller, M. (Eds.). (2001). *From subjects to subjectivities: A handbook of interpretive and participatory methods.* New York: New York University Press.

Ulin, P., Robinson, E. T., & Tolley, E. E. (2005). *Qualitative methods in public health: A field guide for applied research.* San Francisco: Jossey-Bass.

A Selection of Journals That Feature Qualitative and Mixed Methods Studies

Action Research

American Anthropologist

American Journal of Community Psychology

American Journal of Health Promotion

American Journal of Public Health

Australian Journal of Primary Health

Australian and New Zealand Journal of Public Health

Canadian Journal of Public Health

Children, Youth and Environment

Community Mental Health Journal

Culture, Medicine & Psychiatry

Ethnicity & Disease

Ethnicity & Health

Families & Society

Family and Community Health

Field Methods

Forum: Qualitative Social Research (FQSR)

Gateways: International Journal of Community Research and Engagement

Health and Place

Health Education & Behavior

Health Promotion Practice

Health & Social Care in the Community

Human Organization

International Journal of Qualitative Methods

International Journal of Urban Health

Journal of Community Health

Journal of Community Psychology

Journal of Contemporary Ethnography

Journal of Empirical Research on Human Research Ethics

Journal of Health Disparities Research and Practice

Journal of Health and Social Behavior

Journal of Healthcare for Poor and Underserved

Journal of Human Rights Practice

Journal of Mixed Methods Research

Journal of Phenomenological Psychology

Journal of Prevention Practice & Research

Journal of Race, Gender & Class

Journal of the Society for Social Work and Research

Journal of Urban Health

Michigan Journal for Community Service Learning

Progress in Community Health Partnerships

Qualitative Health Research

Qualitative Inquiry

Qualitative Research

Qualitative Social Work

Qualitative Sociology

Social Science & Medicine

Sociological Spectrum

The Qualitative Report

Websites and Other Resources

http://www.nsf.gov/pubs/2004/nsf04219/start.htm (excellent proceedings from workshop on qualitative methods at the National Science Foundation)

http://www.uofaweb.ualberta.ca/iiqm/Conferences.cfm (comprehensive site from the University of Alberta in Canada, which sponsors an international qualitative methods conference annually)

http://obssr.od.nih.gov/pdf/Qualitative.PDF (free downloadable guide to submitting qualitative proposals to the National Institutes of Health)

http://www.scolari.com (information and downloadable software demos for ATLAS.ti, Nud*ist, The Ethnograph, etc.)

http://www.nova.edu/ssss/QR (online journal *The Qualitative Report*)

http://www.nova.edu/ssss/QR/web.html (comprehensive list of web resources for qualitative researchers)

http://www.quarc.de (German–English online resource)

http://qualitative-research.net (German–English–Spanish site with online journal)

http://www.coe.uga.edu/quig (multidisciplinary interest group at the University of Georgia—sponsors national research meeting annually)

http://ejournals.library.ualberta.ca/index.php/IJQM/index (*International Journal of Qualitative Methods*)

http://www.phs.utoronto.ca/qualmethod/ (Centre for Critical Qualitative Health Research at the University of Toronto School of Public Health)

2

Choosing the Right Qualitative Approach(es)

Qualitative methods represent different things to different people. Following is a partial listing illustrating the latter:

Perspectives/Approaches:

- Grounded theory
- Ethnography
- Case study
- Symbolic interactionist
- Narrative
- Constructivist
- Hermeneutic
- Phenomenologic/lifeworld
- Life course
- Feminist
- Participatory action/CBPR

Analytic methods:

- Thematic analysis
- Content analysis
- Case study analysis
- Grounded theory analysis

- Narrative analysis
- Phenomenological analysis
- Conversation analysis
- Discourse analysis

There are a few caveats about this listing. First, the items are neither exhaustive nor mutually exclusive—changes in terminology and general intellectual ferment ensure that any such lists are a work in progress. Second, researchers often mix and match approaches and analytic methods. Some pairings are historically intertwined (e.g., symbolic interactionism and grounded theory), some match up well (e.g., life course perspective and case study analysis), some are more recent mergers (e.g., constructivism and grounded theory), and others are incompatible (e.g., hermeneutic approaches and content analysis). Finally, a few of these analytic methods have a tradition of incorporating quantitative data along with qualitative data (e.g., content analysis, case studies, and ethnography).

This chapter is devoted to six of the most commonly used qualitative approaches: ethnography, grounded theory, case studies, narrative, phenomenological, and community-based participatory research (CBPR) approaches. The choice of which to use is neither formulaic (i.e., if your topic is x, then the qualitative approach must be y), nor is it necessarily confined to one approach. After perusing this chapter, readers are urged to research additional literature on specific methods (see the end of this and subsequent chapters) before making a final decision.

Six Primary Approaches in Qualitative Research

Ethnography

Ethnographic research has been enshrined as a method, a theoretical orientation, and even a philosophical paradigm (Tedlock, 2000). Although its popularity has ebbed and flowed over the years, ethnography has maintained its central position as the quintessential qualitative method. Its reliance on direct observation and *emic* (or insider) perspectives sets a high standard for commitment that stands in contrast to the *etic* (or outsider) perspective assumed by many researchers. In addition to requiring skills in gaining rapport, engaging in intense and ongoing observation, and taking field notes, ethnography implies an attitude or stance. Specifically, it means that one adopts a *holistic perspective*, viewing all aspects of the phenomenon under study as parts of an interrelated whole.

Ethnography also embraces *cultural relativism,* a perspective holding that cultures must be understood on their own terms, not judged by the beliefs and values of other, more powerful cultures (Fetterman, 1989). Although intolerable if taken to the extreme (e.g., considering the Holocaust to be a manifestation of German cultural values that should not be judged by "outsiders"), cultural relativism has value as a challenge to *ethnocentrism,* or the denigration of cultures other than one's own.

Despite its trademark method of participant observation, ethnography does not preclude quantitative data and analyses. Anthropologists have for a long time incorporated measures and statistical analyses in their work (e.g., changes in caloric intake or group differences in social networks).

Heavily influenced by criticism from native peoples and postmodernist self-doubt, ethnography has undergone tremendous change in recent decades. Two distinct trends are notable. First, ethnography became more self-reflexive and intellectually adventurous. Thus, straightforward description of an assumed reality in a faraway culture (with the investigator remaining invisible in the telling) gave rise to deeper interpretations and multiple realities found closer to home. Along the way, ethnography evolved in new directions: on the one hand becoming introspective (giving rise to *autoethnography*), and on the other hand experimenting with new forms of representation (*performance ethnography*). A second trend in ethnography took place on the margins of academia, centered largely in public health and community development. Variously referred to as *applied ethnography* (Chambers, 2000) and *rapid ethnographic assessment* (REA; Manderson & Aaby, 1992), this iteration of the method rendered it time sensitive and resource conserving. REA proved especially useful in global health, in which initiating improvements in sanitation, nutrition, and disease prevention depended on quick turnaround and a respectful interface with local beliefs and practices. Examples include research on nutritional and dietary deficiencies (Scrimshaw & Gleason, 1992) and social and cultural factors influencing the spread of HIV/AIDS (Scrimshaw, Carballo, Ramos, & Blair, 1991). In each of these, the researchers relied on knowledge of the local culture in combination with time-sensitive methods to assess the nature and scope of the problem and its possible resolution.

Doing ethnography means focusing on a cultural system with identifiable features. The boundaries may be physical such as the walls of a hospital or the perimeters of a neighborhood, they may be defined by shared identities (e.g., gang members, transgender sex workers, runaway adolescents), or they may be in cyberspace (Kozinets, 2010). Ethnographic inquiry means operating on several levels simultaneously to infer the tacit rules of the culture or subculture from the myriad actions and interactions being witnessed.

Ethnography clearly has its demands, most notably the amount of time and effort required. Due in part to this intensity, it is less frequently used compared to other options. Nevertheless, ethnography is the progenitor of qualitative methods; its place in the toolkit is secure.

Grounded Theory

Grounded theory (GT) has emerged as one of the most well-known approaches in qualitative research since its debut in the late 1960s (Glaser & Strauss, 1967). Closely aligned with symbolic interactionism and sociology at the Chicago School, GT sparked broad interest among researchers in a variety of disciplines and professions (McKibbon & Gadd, 2004).

GT's systematic demystifying of methods is one of its most attractive features. It has evolved significantly over the years, surviving a dispute between Glaser and Strauss (the latter of whom was joined by Juliet Corbin in subsequent works) and more recently adapted to fit constructivism (Charmaz, 2006) and postmodernism (Clarke, 2005). The popularity and accessibility of GT have undoubtedly led to the wider acceptance of all qualitative methods over the past three decades.

Although subject to variations in practice and in use of terminology (Walker & Myrick, 2006), GT entails inductive coding from the data, memo writing to document analytic decisions, and weaving in theoretical ideas and concepts without permitting them to drive or constrain the study's emergent findings. In an elegant inversion of the theory-driven deduction common to quantitative research, GT has made the pursuit of mid-range theories a respectable, even desirable outcome of qualitative research.

Studies using GT typically involve interviews with a moderately sized sample of carefully selected persons (20 to 30 is about right, but sample sizes can be smaller or larger). Cycling between data collection and analysis, GT begins with *open coding* of interview transcripts. The process of coding may use *sensitizing concepts* drawn from the literature, extant theories, and previous research, but its primary goal is inductive. Coding proceeds to axial and selective phases, gradually creating a parsimonious conceptual framework. Along the way, the researcher employs constant comparative analysis to examine contrasts across respondents, situations, and settings. As will be seen in Chapter 8, the procedures of GT are well-explicated. Although terminology varies, all forms of GT require a good deal of intellectual heavy lifting.

Case Study Analysis

Case studies have a long and honorable history in qualitative research (Feagin, Orum, & Sjoberg, 1991; Stake, 2005; Yin, 2004), and the term is used to refer to approach, method, and product. As studies of "bounded systems of action" (Snow & Anderson, 1991, p. 152), case studies draw on the ability of the qualitative researcher to extract depth and meaning in context. A psychiatric ward, a religious cult, a rural village, or new tobacco legislation can be the focus of a case study. Its goals may be description and analysis of the ethnographic present or of the historic past. Case studies play an important role in program evaluation (Greene, 2000). A study of an exemplary hospice program, for example, can offer insights into best practices with dying patients and their families. Noteworthy events can provide an opportunity to explore historical and social changes (e.g., the 1962 Cuban Missile Crisis or the 1992 Rodney King riots in Los Angeles; Yin, 2004). Eric Klinenberg's *Heat Wave* (2002) used media reports, documents, and interviews to provide a "social autopsy" case study of the disastrous effects of Chicago's 1994 heat wave on the elderly poor. According to Flyvbjerg (2006), case studies can be paradigmatic in their impact, as in the example of Geertz's (1973) groundbreaking analysis of a Balinese cockfight.

Regardless of its subject matter, the case study draws on multiple perspectives and data sources to produce contextually rich and meaningful interpretation. In this regard, it is important to distinguish case studies in qualitative research from their counterparts in clinical education. The latter—a commonly used pedagogical tool for training students—helps illustrate the application of clinical theories in individual cases. In qualitative research, the case study is a method of inquiry for knowledge development that necessitates systematic processes of data collection and analysis (Donmoyer, 1990). Paraphrasing the writings of Thomas Kuhn, Flyvbjerg (2006) notes that "a discipline without a large number of thoroughly executed case studies is a discipline without systematic production of exemplars, and a discipline without exemplars is an ineffective one. In social science, a greater number of good case studies could help remedy this situation" (p. 242).

Case study methods are not as explicitly described as grounded theory and thus leave more analytic discretion to the researcher. This is especially true of multiple case studies in which the challenge is one of aggregating across cases while maintaining the distinctive nature of each case (Campbell & Arens, 1998; Ragin, 1987; Stake, 2005; Yin, 2008). However, when the object(s) of inquiry requires holism over disaggregation, case study analysis is most likely the route to take.

Narrative Approaches

Narrative approaches (NA) have tremendous intuitive appeal given their emphasis on the power of the spoken word (Mishler, 1986; Polkinghorne, 1988). Indeed, their popularity and widespread invocation have led to an indiscriminate use of the term *narrative* for virtually any human utterance (Riessman & Quinney, 2005), extending into therapeutic and self-help domains in which clients are asked to "re-story" their lives (White & Epston, 1990). Our interest is in NA as a diverse set of research methods focusing on how something is said as well as what is said.

Rooted in literature, history, and sociolinguistics, narrative approaches assume that speaking and writing are forms of meaning-making. NA fall into two basic types: (1) *narrative analysis* of interviews designed to elicit storytelling, and (2) *conversation* and *discourse analyses* of naturally occurring speech. Narrative analysis, influenced by William Labov, Elliott Mishler, and Catherine Riessman, uses in-depth interviewing to encourage respondents to talk freely about their lives. Analyses involve repeatedly listening to a tape of the interview and scrutinizing the transcript to identify "stories" from which structural components are then delineated. In addition, the narrative analyst may examine how respondents "voice" themselves and others, thereby indicating social relationships and the meanings attached to them (Sands, 2004).

Naturally occurring conversations are ripe with meaning, whether between friends or virtual strangers. Conversation analysis (CA), with roots in sociology and ethnomethodology (Gubrium & Holstein, 2000; Sacks & Garfinkel, 1970), examines sequencing, turn taking, "holding the floor," interruption, and other aspects of conversation that reveal how social roles and identities are manifested during talk (Farnell & Graham, 2000). Audiotaped transcriptions of conversations between parents and children (or doctors and patients) can be analyzed with CA to offer clues to how interpersonal communication both shapes and reflects social interaction.

Discourse analysis (DA) emerged as a technique for identifying the social meanings reflected in talk and text (Gee, 2005). Meaning can be ascertained from a variety of indices, including choice of words and idioms, speaking rhythm and cadence, inflection, intonation, gestures, and nonverbal utterances (groans, sighs, laughter, etc.). Foucauldian discourse analysis, which draws on Foucault's critiques of hegemonic power and its influence on social meaning-making, tends to operate at a more abstract level than the everyday discourses of interest to most qualitative researchers.

Standing in direct contrast to Foucauldian analyses are the best-selling popular books by sociolinguist Deborah Tannen in which she explores how men and women "just don't understand" one another (1990) and analyzes the volatile communications between mothers and daughters (2006).

Specific techniques for conducting the various narrative approaches differ, but all share a level of immersion that places considerable demands on the researcher. A requirement that the researcher become intensely involved in linguistic structures and meaning also raises concerns about losing the larger social context, although this need not be the case (Gubrium & Holstein, 2000; Riessman, 1993). When properly contextualized, studies of narrative can illuminate the foreground as well as the behind-the-scenes aspects of individual lives, programs, and practice.

Phenomenological Analysis

Phenomenological analysis (PA) explores the lived experience of a phenomenon. PA owes much to the early 20th-century writings of Edmund Husserl and to later developmental work by Giorgi (1985) and Moustakas (1994) in psychology, Benner in health care (1994), and van Manen in education (2002). PA puts the focus on deeper meanings achieved by prolonged immersion. Its use has been heaviest in psychology and nursing.

In PA, the researcher must rely on "bracketing," or sidelining preconceptions about what is real (what Husserl terms "epoche"). Study participants are individuals who share a particular life experience (e.g., cancer survivors, crime victims, adoptive parents). Analyses of interview data are conducted to find the "essence" or common themes in their experiences. Phenomenological findings explore not only what participants experience, but also the situations and conditions of those experiences.

PA interviews, conducted with around 6 to 10 participants, begin with broad, open-ended questioning to ensure the rapport and openness necessary to access the participant's lived experience. Multiple interviews with each participant are needed to achieve needed depth (Creswell, 2007). PA examines interview transcripts in search of quotes and statements that are emblematic in meaning. These are clustered into themes that form the architecture of the findings.

Guidelines for conducting PA are among the least explicit, a reflection of its philosophical origins in which exegesis takes diverse and complex directions (van Manen sponsors a website to help fill this informational gap: www.phenomenologyonline.com). Nevertheless, PA is uniquely suited to leave readers feeling as if they have "walked a mile in the shoes" of participants.

Community-Based Participatory Research

Community-based participatory research (CBPR) has become prominent in public health research (Israel, Eng, Schulz, & Parker, 2005; Minkler & Wallerstein, 2003). Its popularity can be traced to post-1960s movements advocating community empowerment in general (Fals-Borda, 1998; Freire, 1973; Travers, 1997) and power sharing in research in particular (Foster-Fishman, Berkowitz, Lounsbury, Jacobson, & Allen, 2001; Nelson, Ochocka, Griffin, & Lord, 1998). Recent impetus has come from the move away from academic-based, controlled trials to "real world" interventions characteristic of global public health (Leung et al., 2004). The problems associated with experimental trials, often decried as "noise" (Hohmann & Shear, 2002), include low rates of recruitment; high rates of study attrition; and misunderstandings arising from differences in culture, language, and social status. Feasibility and relevance of a study suffer when there is little or no buy-in from a community.

CBPR shares much in common with *action research* and *participatory action research*, which are traceable to the seminal work of Kurt Lewin (1946). What unites these is a fundamental commitment to community empowerment and concerted action in pursuit of social betterment (Reason & Bradbury, 2007; Stringer, 2007). CBPR interprets this commitment to include egalitarian partnerships with community members in which all parties contribute to the research. CBPR may be applied to a de facto "community" of research participants. Pinto (2009), for example, worked with representatives from HIV-prevention organizations as his "community," and Salmon (2007) deployed similar techniques in a study with aboriginal mothers in Western Canada. In the majority of instances, however, the partnership is with a geographically proximal "community," however defined by its members.

CBPR can be seen as embracing "three Ps": It is a *perspective* that ideally infuses a study from start to finish, it connotes a *partnership* of equals among researchers and community participants, and it requires active *participation* by all parties. CBPR partnerships tend to work best when all parties are willing to commit time and resources, but not all partnerships reach the fully egalitarian ideal (Chung & Lounsbury, 2006; Cornwall & Jewkes, 1995).

It is important to note that CBPR is not inherently qualitative—mixed methods or even quantitative-only designs may be pursued. Yet the compatibility of qualitative methods with what CBPR stands for is unarguable, i.e., the additional benefits of rapport building and making research more accessible and acceptable.

In addition to addressing public health problems, CBPR enhances local capacity building (Israel et al., 2005). With optimal application, a CBPR study brings resources both financial (salaries for research staff, payments of incentives) and in human capital (education and training in research skills such as interviewing, use of computers and software, organizational leadership). Because of its prolonged commitment, CBPR typically lasts not weeks but years, its partnerships evolving as new public health problems emerge and the existing infrastructure is reinvigorated to meet these challenges.

CBPR has been a valuable tool in the fight against HIV/AIDS, in cancer prevention, in combating neighborhood crime, and in addressing environmental health hazards (Israel et al., 2005; Minkler & Wallerstein, 2003). Projects may involve needs assessments, health promotion campaigns, civic and political activism, or program evaluation. Clearly, not all research topics point to CBPR, nor should all researchers undertake it. It takes a very committed and socially conscious investigative team to subordinate their collective egos to the wishes of the community.

Box 2.1	**CBPR and Cancer: Making Innovative Use of a Public Library System**

One of the more innovative uses of CBPR in urban settings has been the Queens Library HealthLink Project (QLHP) led by psychologist Bruce Rapkin and colleagues at the Einstein College of Medicine and Montefiore Medical Center in New York City. Funded by the National Cancer Institute, the QLHP uses a participatory research approach to reducing racial and ethnic disparities in cancer by using public library branches as a base for outreach to surrounding neighborhoods. Trained public health specialists collaborate in health education, data gathering, and implementation of health-promotion projects in cooperation with local hospitals and clinics. Such projects, ranging from quilting parties to health fairs, draw on cancer survivors and other volunteers to raise awareness and enhance community cohesion. A central focus of

(Continued)

(Continued)

the QLHP was the formation of Cancer Action Councils (CACs) made up of community members from diverse organizations. The ultimate goal of the QLHP is to ensure sustainable CACs that will continue to work in spreading awareness about cancer prevention and early detection. As one way of monitoring the impact of the project, street intercept surveys are regularly conducted to assess rates of cancer screening, smoking, cancer awareness, and so forth. Perhaps not surprisingly, there are challenges along the way, including language barriers and the fears of undocumented immigrants. More insulated ethnic enclaves are harder to reach, as are young people. Nevertheless, the project has brought benefits not only in health awareness but also in fostering a spirit of communal belonging. As one CAC member said in an interview, "I never want to see the CAC go away."

Commentary: The Queens Library System, one of the largest in the United States, offers an unusual yet highly efficient model that piggybacks upon an extensive network of public facilities. Although the formation and maintenance of the CACs entail far more sustained effort than a purely top-down endeavor (such as a media campaign), the benefits are more likely to be multifaceted and deeply rooted in community priorities and values.

Constructivist and Critical Theory Influences

The aforementioned descriptions are of methods with distinct features and procedures, all deeply rooted in philosophy, linguistics, and the social sciences. As noted in Chapter 1, several have subsequently been affected by the rise of constructivism and the paradigm debates that ensued after the 1980s. Presented as a fully developed (and superior) replacement for positivism (Denzin & Lincoln, 2005; Lincoln & Guba, 1985), the constructivist movement introduced a degree of self-consciousness about epistemology not seen before (Morgan, 2007).

The embrace of constructivism and critical theories depended on the persuasiveness of their applications and by the degree of fit with each method. Narrative and phenomenological approaches had little distance to travel in this regard with their predisposition toward social construction and reflexivity. As noted earlier in this chapter, ethnography proved to be a ripe target for change as it shifted "from participant observation to the observation of participation" (Tedlock, 2000, p. 465).

Multiple genres flowered, including critical ethnography (Kincheloe & McLaren, 2000; Madison, 2005), autoethnography (Ellis & Bochner, 2000), performance ethnography (McCall, 2000), feminist ethnography (Tedlock, 2000), and so on.

Annells (1996) and Mills, Bonner, and Francis (2006) find a strong constructivist thread running through grounded theory (even though it is usually the winner in the category of "qualitative method most likely to be post-positivist"). Critical theory is also compatible with GT. Cooney (2006), for example, combined critical theory epistemology and grounded theory methods to analyze data from focus group interviews with Spanish- and English-speaking low-income families. A well-articulated version of constructivist grounded theory has been developed by Charmaz (2006). Charmaz distinguishes constructivist from objectivist grounded theory, noting that the former relies on interpretive frames and the latter focuses on explanation and prediction. Given the flexibility and neutrality of grounded theory—it predates and transcends the paradigm debates— such an adaptation extends rather than breaks with tradition. CBPR has strong foundations in pragmatism and utility as they relate to solving real-life problems (Levin & Greenwood, 2001). Yet constructivist iterations of CBPR have emerged. Eng and colleagues (2005), for example, cite constructivism as their research paradigm in working with rural African American communities in North Carolina.

Critical theories are typically attached to whatever methodology is appropriate for the study's goals, quantitative or qualitative. Ford and Airhihenbuwa (2010) link critical race theory to public health research, asserting that this connection is necessary to fully explore the meaning of health disparities.

Mixing and Matching Qualitative Approaches

The risk of specifying six (or any number of) qualitative approaches lies in conveying a message of discreteness that belies the blurriness of definitions and applications in qualitative inquiry. Some case studies, for example, are hard to distinguish from ethnographies because both adopt an in-depth holistic perspective. Meanwhile, qualitative researchers may deliberately mix and match qualitative approaches to find the right combination (not to be confused with mixing qualitative and quantitative methods, the subject of Chapter 3). This occurs within two plausible scenarios: (1) a fusion or hybrid approach, or (2) a juxtaposition of two approaches side by side or in sequence. Annells (2006) refers to this as "turning the prism" via theoretical and methodological triangulation (p. 59).

Matters get complicated when considering (1) the different points at which mixing may occur—from interpretive paradigm to overall approach to specific method of analysis; and (2) the extent to which one is concerned about paradigm and method congruence. Cross-paradigm mixing has been disparaged as incommensurable (Lincoln & Guba, 2000), although not everyone agrees with this contention.

A good example of this can be found in the groundbreaking work of Newman, Fox, Roth, and Mehta (2004) in which they used a side-by-side paradigm approach to study school shootings in Kentucky and Arkansas (predating the Columbine and Virginia Tech tragedies). Newman and colleagues used both positivist and interpretivist lenses, drawing on "factual" data from forensic analyses and court records and also analyzing transcripts of interviews that provided conflicting (and conflicted) accounts by students, school staff, and parents of the shooters as well as the victims.

Although less common (and much more likely to be deployed at the analysis stage), hybrid mixing is described by Fereday and Muir-Cochrane (2006) in their blending of the inductive procedures of Boyatzis (1998) with "template style" coding (Crabtree & Miller, 1999) to study nursing performance. Similarly, Wilson and Hutchison (1991) propose the side-by-side use of phenomenology and grounded theory as complementary and mutually enriching perspectives.

In an example of mixing in sequence, Teram, Schachter, and Stalker (2005) conducted grounded theory interviews with female survivors of childhood sexual abuse enrolled in physical therapy, then shifted to "pragmatic action research" to transform the analyses and findings via working groups of participants and physical therapists. The groups' joint production of a handbook for health professionals created a more sensitive set of guidelines for working with abuse survivors.

A few related caveats are pertinent here. First, incongruities can bring complications during the mixing of qualitative approaches. Phenomenological analyses of grounded theory interviews would be likely to suffer from the lack of deep attunement to meaning and lived experience (Wimpenny & Gass, 2000). Second, mixing carries the risk of "method slurring" (Baker, Wuest, & Stern, 1992) wherein one or both approaches lose their integrity and capacity to make a contribution. This is obviously a greater problem for hybrid than for juxtaposing formats.

Last but not least, unsuccessful attempts at mixing (i.e., method slurring) point to the widespread use of generic qualitative methods, particularly in the applied professions (Caelli, Ray, & Mill, 2003). The lack of paradigm and method allegiance posed by a generic approach raises concerns about producing a watered-down and non-rigorous product, thereby losing the integrity of the original methods (Sandelowski & Barroso, 2002). While arguing against generic approaches is not likely to make them go away, demonstrating an awareness of their limitations and seeking ways to enhance the study's credibility and rigor can help to offset their limitations.

Qualitative Methods in Program Evaluation

Qualitative evaluation has a long history, especially in the field of education (Bogdan & Taylor, 1975; Cook & Reichardt, 1979; Fetterman, 1989; Guba & Lincoln, 1981, 1989; Patton, 2002; Stake, 1995). Relying solely on quantitative methods risks losing an understanding of what is happening below the surface (where many an intervention succeeds or fails in ways unbeknownst to the investigator; Padgett, 2009b). It also places enormous trust in quantitative measures of sensitive, fluctuating, and elusive phenomena.

Any number of hidden effects may occur. A program may be found successful, but not for the reasons assumed. It may appear to be a failure according to some outcome measures even though it might have been deemed a success by different methods. Narrow conceptualizations of "success" (e.g., use of a needle exchange) may overlook what clients value more (e.g., access to drug rehabilitation programs). Positive outcomes may be an artifact of biased sampling or measurement error rather than "reality." A clinically tested treatment that succeeds under controlled conditions may fall apart when transplanted to a program beset by scarce resources, a demoralized staff, and unhappy clientele. These concerns point to the need for contextual methods sensitive enough to capture what is happening behind the scenes, not just on the stage.

Summary and Concluding Thoughts

This chapter introduced six primary approaches in qualitative inquiry— ethnography, grounded theory, case studies, phenomenological analysis, narrative approaches, and community-based participatory research—as a menu of options for the qualitative researcher. Not always willing to settle for just one, researchers often mix and match approaches to achieve the most suitable combination for their needs. The topic of interest and the goals of the study drive such choices. Constructivist iterations have also emerged and are especially well developed in grounded theory. Novice researchers are well advised to read specialized texts and articles using these varied approaches to get a sense of how investigators make the most of what each has to offer. Qualitative inquiry is steeped in choices and decisions—a qualitative study can be seen as a series of critical junctures in which the decision trail is rarely, if ever, foreordained. To close out this chapter, Box 2.2 below gives a brief overview of which approaches were used in the NYSS.

Box 2.2   Qualitative Approaches in the New York Services Study

The central goal of the NYSS—to learn about the service system from the users' perspectives—pointed to an interview-dominant study, but this still left several options in choice of qualitative approaches. In Phase 1 of the study, we settled on grounded theory and case study analyses of life history interviews. Grounded theory was selected because we wanted to build an inductive theory or model explaining participants' experiences with homeless, mental health, and substance abuse services. This model, in turn, was meant to inform the study's Phase 2. Case study analysis was necessary in order to have a holistic view of each participant's life. Both approaches were carried over into Phase 2 but with several modifications. In this second phase, participants consisted of 80 new enrollees in four homeless services programs for adults in New York City. Phase 2 interviews with clients consisted of three in-depth interviews over 12 months of follow-up. Baseline interviews were coded using GT. The two follow-up interviews used a template format in which open-ended questions were structured about domains. For these, we used Boyatzis's (1998) method of thematic development, as it was more suitable for the data. Phenomenological and narrative approaches were not used in the NYSS as they were not considered a good fit. We periodically regretted the absence of ethnography, however. Observation was considered to be too time-consuming given the study's priorities, but there were occasions when participants invited us to accompany them in daily activities or when we wished we could observe the agencies in their day-to-day operations. Action or community-based participatory approaches held great appeal but were well beyond the scope and feasibility of the study.

1. Go to Google Scholar or use your college/university access to public health and related journals (see listing in Chapter 1) and locate examples of studies representing each of the six types of qualitative methods presented in this chapter. Download and print an article and bring it to class for discussion.

2. Choose a topic of interest and consult the listing of approaches and techniques at the beginning of this chapter. What combination of these is the best fit for your study?

3. How would you describe the strengths and limitations of each of the six approaches presented in this chapter?

4. Consider the many options possible in mixing among the six qualitative approaches. Discuss in class which appear most (and least) suitable for mixing.

Additional Readings

Ethnography

Agar, M. H. (1980). *The professional stranger: An informal introduction to ethnography.* New York: Academic Press.

DeWalt, K. M., & DeWalt, B. R. (2001). *Participant observation: A guide for fieldworkers.* Walnut Creek, CA: AltaMira Press.

Emerson, R. M. (2001). *Contemporary field research.* Long Grove, IL: Waveland Press.

Fetterman, D. M. (2010). *Ethnography: Step-by-step* (3rd ed.). Thousand Oaks, CA: Sage.

Hammersley, M., & Atkinson, P. (2007). *Ethnography: Principles in practice* (3rd ed.). New York: Routledge.

Kozinets, R. V. (2010). *Netography: Doing ethnographic research online.* Thousand Oaks, CA: Sage.

LeCompte, M. D., & Schensul, J. J. (2010). *Designing and conducting ethnographic research* (2nd ed.) (*Ethnographer's toolkit*, Book 1). Walnut Creek, CA: AltaMira Press.

Lofland, J., & Lofland, L. (1995). *Analyzing social settings: A guide to qualitative observation and analysis* (3rd ed.), Belmont, CA: Wadsworth.

Madison, D. S. (2005). *Critical ethnography* (2nd ed.). Thousand Oaks, CA: Sage.

Grounded Theory

Charmaz, C. (2006). *Constructing grounded theory: A practical guide through qualitative analysis.* Thousand Oaks, CA: Sage.

Corbin, J., & Strauss, A. L. (2008). *Basics of qualitative research* (3rd ed.). Thousand Oaks, CA: Sage.

Dey, I. (1999). *Grounding grounded theory.* San Diego: Academic Press.

Glaser, B. G. (1992). *Basics of grounded theory.* Mill Valley, CA: The Sociology Press.

Glaser, B. G., & Strauss, A. L. (1967). *The discovery of grounded theory.* Chicago: Aldine.

Case Study Analysis

Ragin, C. C., & Becker, H. S. (Eds.). (1992). *What is a case? Exploring the foundations of social inquiry.* Cambridge, UK: Cambridge University Press.

Stake, R. E. (1995). *The art of case study research.* Thousand Oaks, CA: Sage.

Stake, R. E. (2005). *Multiple case study analysis.* New York: Guilford Press.

Yin, R. K. (Ed.). (2004). *The case study anthology.* Thousand Oaks, CA: Sage.

Yin, R. K. (2008). *Case study research: Design and methods* (4th ed.). Thousand Oaks, CA: Sage.

Phenomenology

Benner, P. (Ed.). (1994). *Interpretive phenomenology: Embodiment, caring, and ethics in health and illness.* Thousand Oaks, CA: Sage.

Colaizzi, P. F. (1978). Psychological research as the phenomenologist views it. In R. Valle & M. King (Eds.), *Existential-phenomenological alternatives for psychology* (pp. 48–71). New York: Oxford University Press.

Giorgi, A. (Ed.). (1985). *Phenomenology and psychological research.* Pittsburgh, PA: Duquesne University Press.

Moustakas, C. (1994). *Phenomenological research methods.* Thousand Oaks, CA: Sage.

Polkinghorne, D. E. (1989). Phenomenological research methods. In R. S. Valle & S. Halling (Eds.), *Existential-phenomenological alternatives for psychology* (pp. 41–60). New York: Plenum.

Smith, J. A. (2009). *Interpretive phenomenological analysis: Theory, method, and research.* Thousand Oaks, CA: Sage.

Van Manen, J. (1990). *Researching lived experience: Human science for an action sensitive pedagogy.* Albany: State University of New York Press.

Narrative Approaches

Clandinin, D. J. (Ed.). (2006). *Handbook of narrative inquiry: Mapping a methodology.* Thousand Oaks, CA: Sage.

Cortazzi, M. (1993). *Narrative analysis.* London: Falmer Press.

Gee, J. P. (2005). *An introduction to discourse analysis: Theory and method.* London: Routledge.

Josselson, R., & Lieblich, A. (Eds.). (1999). *Making meaning of narratives* (Vol. 6). Thousand Oaks, CA: Sage.

Riessman, C. K. (1993). *Narrative analysis.* Newbury Park, CA: Sage.

Riessman, C. K. (2008). *Narrative methods for the human sciences.* Thousand Oaks, CA: Sage.

Ten Have, P. (1999). *Doing conversation analysis.* London: Sage.

Action and Community-Based Participatory Research

Cornwall, A., & Jewkes, R. (1995). What is participatory research? *Social Science & Medicine, 41*(12), 1667–1676.

Israel, B. A., Eng, E., Schulz, A. J., & Parker, E. A. (Eds.). (2005). *Methods in community-based participatory research for health.* San Francisco: Jossey-Bass.

Jones, L., & Wells, K. (2007). Strategies for academic and clinician engagement in community-based partnered research. *Journal of the American Medical Association, 297*(4), 407–410.

Minkler, M., & Wallerstein, N. (Eds.). (2003). *Community-based participatory research for health.* San Francisco: Jossey-Bass.

Reason, P., & Bradbury, H. (2007). *The SAGE handbook of action research* (2nd ed.). Thousand Oaks, CA: Sage.

Stringer, E. T. (2007). *Action research: A handbook for practitioners* (3rd ed.). Thousand Oaks, CA: Sage.

Journals Publishing CBPR

Public Health:

American Journal of Health Behavior

American Journal of Public Health

Canadian Journal of Public Health

Cancer Control

Environmental Health Perspectives

Health Education and Behavior

Health Promotion International

Health Promotion Practice

International Journal of Circumpolar Health

Journal of Public Health Management and Practice

Journal of Studies on Alcohol

Public Health

Public Health Nursing

Community Health:

American Journal of Community Psychology

Ethnicity & Disease

Journal of Community Health

Journal of Epidemiology and Community Health

Journal of Urban Health

Progress in Community Health Partnerships: Research, Education, and Action

Medicine:

American Journal of Preventive Medicine

Annals of Family Medicine

Journal of General Internal Medicine

Preventive Medicine

Social Science & Medicine

3

Mixed Methods

The "new era" of method integration (Tashakkori & Creswell, 2007, p. 3) can be seen as a pragmatic response on the part of researchers wanting to maximize their understanding of a particular problem (Johnson & Onwuegbuzie, 2004; Morgan, 2007). Some research topics (such as public opinions about childhood vaccines) are manifestly quantitative; others (such as IV drug users' needle-sharing practices) are undoubtedly qualitative. In the vast middle ground lie many opportunities to use both approaches for synergistic ends.

At the same time, mixed methods designs are complicated and sometimes messy affairs (Creswell & Plano Clark, 2010). Integrating the quantitative and qualitative "sides" poses epistemological and logistical challenges that few research courses address (Tashakkori & Teddlie, 2010). That said, the momentum behind this trend is unlikely to slow down anytime soon.

The Rise of Mixed Methods and Their Rationale(s)

Just as the term *qualitative methods* came of age in the 1970s, *mixed methods* is a fairly recent addition to the research lexicon (Tashakkori & Teddlie, 2010). Formerly (and sometimes still) referred to as "multimethod," "multistrategy," or "triangulation by method," mixed methods studies currently offer a wide and at times confusing array of options (Bryman, 2006; Creswell, 2007; Tashakkori & Teddlie, 2010).

Ethnographers and others have a long history of including quantitative data and analyses. This unheralded "mixing" lost favor as the methods became more interview-based with the rise of grounded theory and narrative approaches. In addition, mixing on the qualitative side was derogated in critiques asserting the incompatibility of positivist assumptions of realism with constructivist assumptions of multiple interpretations (Lincoln & Guba, 1985; Morgan, 2007).

On the quantitative side, the soaring dominance of quantification and statistics by the mid-20th century cast doubt on the value of qualitative data with its small samples and presumed lack of generalizability. Pioneering quantitative methodologists (D. T. Campbell & Stanley, 1963; Cook & Campbell, 1979) acknowledged the utility of qualitative data, but only in a supplementary or minor role. Interestingly, D. T. Campbell (1979) recanted his earlier criticisms of case studies and went further to state that conflicting results in mixed methods studies should cast the quantitative results as suspect "until the reasons for the discrepancy are well understood" (p. 52).

Caracelli and Greene (1997) discuss three reasons for carrying out mixed methods studies, which include triangulation, complementarity, and expansion. *Triangulation,* the earliest and most widely invoked of rationales, refers to comparisons for purposes of corroboration (Morse, 1991). Because triangulation presumes a fixed point of reference waiting to be converged upon, its use has been criticized as naïve and sometimes misleading. It also raises questions when findings are divergent rather than convergent (Flick, 2004; Sandelowski, 2000). *Complementarity* refers to enhancement or clarification. Thus, the quantitative and qualitative substudies represent different pieces of the puzzle. *Expansion* refers to presenting "side-by-side" or juxtaposed findings to keep them intact (Caracelli & Greene, 1997).

Types of Mixed Methods Research

All research designs operate from a premise of intentionality, and mixed methods designs point to the desire to link or integrate. As such, they portend specific procedures to carry this out (Haase & Myers, 1988). Interestingly, few mixed methods studies in the published literature use the terminology and notational systems promulgated by leaders in the field (Creswell, 2007; Morse, 1991; Tashakkori & Teddlie, 2010). Nevertheless, it helps to recognize the many options and approach them in a systematic way. As shown in Table 3.1, the options in designing a mixed methods study involve two primary axes—sequential versus concurrent and dominant/subdominant versus equal (Creswell, 2003; Miller & Fredericks, 2006). *Dominant* refers to which method is given more weight and prominence in the study. When examining a study's written report, this can be glaringly obvious or deeply ambiguous, depending on the study's design and how clearly it is described. *Sequential versus concurrent axes* refers to the timing of the methods, whether used one at a time or simultaneously.

Table 3.1   Mixed Methods Designs Arranged by Timing and Dominance

	Sequential	Concurrent
Dominant–Less Dominant	CELL 1 QUAL → quan qual → QUAN QUAN → qual quan → QUAL	CELL 2—*"Nested"* QUAL + quan QUAN + qual
Equal Weighting	CELL 4 QUAL → QUAN QUAN → QUAL	CELL 3 —*"Fully Integrated"* QUAL + QUAN

Using established notations of capital letters (for dominance or priority), arrows (for sequencing), and plus signs (for simultaneity; Morse, 1991), Table 3.1 shows various possibilities for the sequential and concurrent designs. As might be expected, QUAN-dominant designs are more common than QUAL-dominant designs and dominant/less-dominant designs are more common than equally weighted designs. Both of these observations are a reflection of the way the research world is organized and the tendency to conserve resources and/or favor one method over another. A caveat before we go further: These design types are offered primarily as a heuristic device. In practice, mixed methods studies are complicated and not so easily categorized (Miller & Fredericks, 2006).

Sequential Designs

In sequential designs, how the study's segments are prioritized and integrated depends on its priorities. As shown in Cells 1 and 4 of Table 3.1, this can occur in six different ways. Among the dominant/less-dominant designs, the most common (qual→QUAN and QUAN→qual) typically involve using focus groups or individual interviews to prepare for the "main event" (survey, instrument development, experimental trial, etc.) or to better understand it after the fact. The ecological validity of a quantitative study can be enhanced considerably by grounding the study in qualitative interviews and observation before or after. Conducting focus groups with students and teachers before implementing a safe-sex education program is one example of this approach; positioning the focus groups afterward is another example, albeit for a different purpose.

QUAL→quan and quan→QUAL studies position their quantitative segments as less dominant. An example of the first would be an intensive qualitative case study of an innovative program for individuals with multiple sclerosis that is used to develop questions for a brief online survey of agencies serving MS patients. In the reverse sequence (quan→QUAL), a telephone survey of parents in a school district might be used to select a subsample willing to be interviewed in depth about their experiences with the district's new program on childhood obesity.

Although less common, equal weighting in sequential designs (Cell 4 of Table 3.1) means that both qualitative and quantitative segments receive sufficient allocations of resources to meet their respective sampling and data quality needs.

Concurrent Designs

In concurrent designs, one method may be dominant over the other (QUAN+qual or QUAL+quan) or they may be given equal weight (QUAN+QUAL). As mentioned earlier, "dominant/less dominant" or nested designs (Cell 2 of Table 3.1) are much more common (Creswell, 2007). Box 3.1 offers an example of a QUAN+qual study carried out in different nations.

Box 3.1 A Mixed Methods Study (QUAN+qual) Testing a Measure of Social Capital in Peru and Vietnam

Mixed methods have an intrinsic appeal for instrument development and testing because most measures' underlying constructs are complex and open to differing meanings and interpretations. One such concept, that of *social capital*, has become widely used as an indication of the ways that social relationships may confer health benefits, from fostering a sense of belonging to providing links to valuable resources. The measurement of social capital at the individual level is seen as a potential indicator of health in general and access to health care in particular (Szreter & Woolcock, 2004). DeSilva and colleagues (2006) developed a measure of social capital (the SASCAT), translated it into Spanish and Vietnamese, and administered it to a large sample of children's caregivers (3,000 in Peru and 2,771 in Vietnam). In addition to psychometric tests of the measure's validity, the researchers criterion-sampled 20 Peruvian and 24 Vietnamese respondents for in-depth interviews. These "cognitive interviews," lasting from 1 to 2 hours, elicited further thoughts and ideas related to each SASCAT item. An example of an item is, "In the past 12 months, have you joined together with other community members to address a common problem or issue?" The interviews were audiotaped and content analyzed to see if (and how often) open-ended comments diverged from the authors' original intention regarding each item's meaning. The findings were revealing. Although the quantitative factor analysis results from the two countries were strikingly similar, the qualitative interviews brought several cultural misunderstandings to the surface. The concept of "community," for example, was readily accepted in Vietnam but not understood by many Peruvians (who defined it as one's social support network, not the surrounding area). In both Peru and Vietnam, "trust" was not considered something one can impute to the "community" in general but only to known individuals. Similarly, "help from others" was largely defined as economic support—contrary to the measure's inclusion of emotional support within the definition. The authors understandably concluded that cognitive validation needs to precede instrument development.

Commentary: This study's QUAN+qual design was an ambitious and successful application of mixed methods. The two methods were used for corroboration as well as completeness (i.e., the researchers did not posit a single meaning for each item but instead sought out multiple meanings to improve the measure). The findings demonstrate the critical importance of qualitative methods in cross-cultural research in which subjective meanings can vary along cultural lines. If this is not taken into consideration, quantitative data collection will be prone to error and misunderstandings.

In QUAN+qual designs, researchers typically collect qualitative data to enliven or illustrate their quantitative findings, for example, excerpts from responses to open-ended questions or case vignettes (Morgan, 1997). In the reverse QUAL+quan approach, qualitative researchers might collect some quantitative data via standardized measures or they might use supplementary quantitative data from documents or archives. Snow and Anderson (1991) made use of tracking data from various agencies to supplement their intensive interviews and ethnographic observation of the homeless. The resulting depictions contained both statistical and ethnographic descriptions of their lives. Using quantitative data can be risky with small samples, but if done judiciously it need not detract from the inductive, emergent nature of a qualitative study. Similarly, the inclusion of ancillary qualitative data does not challenge the primacy of a "big QUAN" study. A QUAL+QUAN study (Cell 3) is among the rarest of mixed methods types due to aforementioned demands on time and resources as well as the challenges of fully integrating the two "sides."

Mixed Methods: Ways of Going About It

Structural and Design Decisions: What, When, Where, and How?

Leaving the abstract realm of design types for real-world decisions about mixing methods requires that we unravel the research process and decide which phases will (or should) intersect and which will remain intact. Are there constraints on doing this, or can one mix and match at will? Consider the following series of statements:

- Paradigms (post-positivist, constructivist, critical) do not dictate methods (grounded theory, phenomenological, experimental/quantitative, surveys, etc.).
- Methods do not dictate data collection techniques (interviews, question-naires, observation).
- Techniques of data collection do not dictate data analyses.

Such assertions are strongly opposed by postmodern contentions that one cannot mix positivist and constructivist epistemologies (Lincoln & Guba, 2000). But such objections have not slowed the movement toward mixing below the paradigmatic level (Morgan, 2007). (The reader might want to return to Figure 1.1 in Chapter 1 on page 15, which shows the downward line or spiral of a study.) Thus, a grounded theory study can be carried out using post-positivist or constructivist epistemologies; some studies appear to do both simultaneously. At a lower level, many a study has transformed qualitative data into numbers. To be sure, some combinations do not work, for example, narrative analysis and quantitative data. Moreover, one should not mix and match willy-nilly without considerations of fit and appropriateness.

According to Sandelowski (2000), most mixing takes place "on the shop floor of research" (p. 246) during sampling, data collection, and data analysis. Tashakkori and Creswell (2007) discuss dual dimensions to sampling (probability and purposive), data collection (quantitative and qualitative), data analysis (statistical and thematic), and presentation of the findings (numeric and narrative).

The points of contact between the quantitative and qualitative sides can be many or few. Sequential designs leave open the opportunity for each substudy to remain intact (assuming a reasonable connection is made). In concurrent designs, the parallel processes, or "strands" (Tashakkori & Creswell, 2007, p. 3), may intersect at one or more phases. The lowest level of mixing intensity is when the two sides stay separate and come together only at the end when findings are juxtaposed.

Mixing at the data analysis level, according to Tashakkori and Teddlie (2010), may include "qualitizing" quantitative data and its opposite process of "quantitizing" qualitative data. The latter of these, which refers to converting qualitative data into numbers or variables, has a long history in content analysis. (An example of "quantitizing" is provided in Box 3.2.) Sandelowski (2000) "qualitized" her quantitative data by creating profiles or categorical types from scores on standardized measures.

Box 3.2	"Quantitizing" Data in a Grounded Theory Study of Breast and Prostate Cancer Online Discussion Boards

Online chat rooms and discussion boards offer an abundance of narrative data for qualitative analysis. Gooden and Winefield (2007) used grounded theory and a "quasi-numeric" (p. 103) approach to examine gender differences in language styles and communication among cancer survivors communicating online. They started with a hypothesis positing greater use of emotional communications by women and greater use of informational communications by men. They examined online communications among 69 women with breast cancer and 77 men with prostate cancer by using open, axial, and selective coding

(Continued)

(Continued)

conducted independently by two readers. The number of codes per message (or posting) and the frequency with which individuals posted were calculated and displayed in tables in the published article. From these analyses, two selective codes ("information support" and "emotional support") were identified along with their respective axial and open codes. Examples of axial codes included "facts about the disease" (under information support) and "coping philosophies" (under emotional support). Instances of open codes were counted in each database and categorized proportionately under each of these two main headings. As a result, Gooden and Winefield found that information communication comprised 60% of women's communications and 64% of men's communications. Thus, there were modest (and probably non-significant) gender differences in the frequency of emotional (versus informational) communication. Virtually all of the results section of the article was devoted to describing the codes, thereby revealing subtle but meaningful aspects of gender. Under "information support," for example, men were likely to offer detailed factual information compared to briefer informational summaries supplied by women. Under "emotional support," women used warm dialogue and affectionate phrasing, while men suggested to their peers that they "keep their chin up" and "beat the bastard." In other code domains, such as use of humor and group spirit, men and women did not differ.

Commentary: This study's use of a hypothesis and a QUAL+quan design set the stage for the "quantitizing" that followed. However, the quantitative findings comparing men and women were modest and anticlimactic. In the study's write-up, the numbers told a small story, but the qualitative themes and interpretations were the main event.

Box 3.3	**The Difficulty in Ascertaining Research Designs in Mixed Methods: An Example From a Study of Rural Bangladeshi Couples and Pregnancy Termination**

Few published reports of mixed methods studies use the typologies and design notations described in this chapter. Journal reviewers are not likely to demand them, and the complexities of mixing methods do not always map onto extant typologies. A mixed methods study published in the *American Journal of Public*

Health in 2008 offers a case in point. In the article, the authors Gipson and Hindin report using mixed methods to understand how rural Bangladeshi couples make family planning decisions including pregnancy termination. To do so, they draw upon health survey and surveillance data from 3,052 couples as well as 84 in-depth interviews conducted with 19 couples. Quantitative survey questions about childbearing and pregnancy termination were a key interest in the qualitative interviews, but the investigators used a life history technique in the latter to avoid appearing intrusive or invading of the couples' privacy.

Although the authors do not say, the design appears to be sequential in that the quantitative data came from surveys (conducted from 1998 to 2003), and the qualitative purposive sample was drawn from a roster of couples who were enrolled in the survey as of 2004. On the other hand, the study design could be seen as concurrent since it juxtaposes the two "sides" without reference to the time lapse rather than presents them as temporally separate.

It is also difficult to decide whether the design is dominant or equally weighted. It appears to be QUAN-dominant, since the findings section gives full coverage to the statistical analyses in tabular and text format followed by reference to the qualitative findings with selected illustrative quotes. The size and volume of the quantitative data, combined with a foreshortened qualitative data analysis (described by Gipson and Hindin [2008] as "focused" [p. 1828]), reinforces this notion of QUAN-dominance. However, this scenario is not entirely borne out in the weight the authors give to the two sides while discussing the findings and their implications. For example, the qualitative results offer insightful perspectives on a number of topics including the stigma of having a child when the older children are nearing marital age (thereby hurting the older children's marital prospects), the use of traditional forms of abortifacients such as roots and homeopathic tablets, and the hidden ways that women terminate pregnancy without telling their husbands. All of these were the result of multiple in-depth interviews conducted with husbands and wives separately. It is hard to imagine how surveys could have brought forth such deeply sensitive information.

With regard to the "what" question, Bryman (2006) reports that the concurrent mixing of standardized surveys and qualitative interviews is most common, the latter often based on a purposively selected subsample from the larger survey sample. From the qualitative side, focus groups are a popular choice for mixing; life history interviews and ethnographic observation are less amenable to mixing. From the quantitative side, randomized clinical trials offer less fit for mixed methods compared to standardized interviews and surveys.

Some Examples of Mixed Methods Studies

The following are a few iterations of mixed methods designs with hypothetical examples.

- *A sequential design in which scores on an instrument administered during a survey are subsequently used for criterion sampling of a small subsample for qualitative interviews.* For example, a study of depression in college students might use scores on the depressive symptom scale to identify students at highest and lowest risk. These students could then be interviewed in depth about their college experiences and life stressors.
- *A concurrent design at the data collection stage in which in-depth interviews are paired with Likert-type survey questions.* For example, a study of South African women might administer measures of exposure to partner violence in a community meeting along with post-meeting focus groups for volunteers willing to discuss the issue at greater length.
- *A concurrent design at the data analysis stage in which qualitative data are "quantitized" and converted to categorical variables and tested using statistical analysis.* In the NYSS, for example, we conducted case study analyses and categorized participants by whether they were "users" vs. "non-users" of drugs and alcohol during their year-long participation in the study. This dichotomous yes/no variable was the outcome in a series of logistic regression analyses comparing individuals grouped by race, housing status, gender, and so on (Padgett, Stanhope, Henwood, & Stefancic, 2011). Although our sample size was fairly large for a qualitative study (N = 75) and enabled use of multivariate analyses, smaller-scale studies might use bivariate analyses or non-parametric statistics such as Fisher's exact test.
- *A sequential design in which quantitative data are "qualitized" (i.e., statistical analyses are used to produce profiles or clusters that set the stage for qualitative interviews with study participants within each cluster to corroborate these analyses).* A standardized interview of gay male adolescents might, for example, be used to create a typology of HIV risk based on the scores on measures of substance abuse, depression, and social support. Respondents who fit the "high risk" profile could be interviewed in depth and contrasted with those who fit the "low risk."
- *A longitudinal concurrent design in which the quantitative and qualitative sides mutually inform one another.* An example is shown in Figure 3.1 for a hypothetical community-based intervention. As shown, focus groups with key stakeholders in the community help guide the content for a household needs assessment survey. Findings from the survey help shape the intervention (e.g., a nutrition program for low-income parents) that is pilot-tested and then implemented. Throughout the intervention, ethnographic observation is used to help evaluate process and fidelity aspects of the implementation, identify problem areas, and collect data from participants (children, parents, school officials) assessing effectiveness. Depending on the study's aims, the ethnographic data may be confined to informing the quantitative work, or it may be separately presented as findings and compared (or triangulated) with the quantitative outcome data.

- *A longitudinal sequential design oscillating between the quantitative and qualitative sides.* In contrast to the previous example, this design involves alternating between sides over time. As depicted in Figure 3.2, such oscillation could take the form of ethnographic observations on an American Indian reservation that are used to inform a community survey on needs of children and families. The survey's findings then lead to criterion-sampled focus groups of adolescents, the results of which inform a targeted intervention to prevent adolescent suicide.

Figure 3.1   A Longitudinal Mixed Methods Design

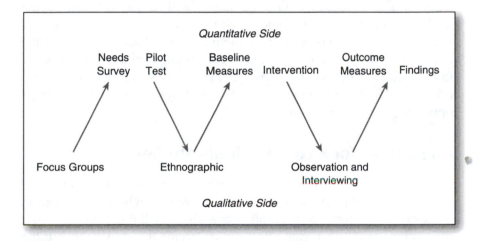

Figure 3.2   An Oscillating Mixed Methods Design

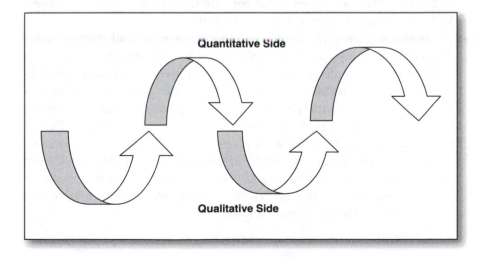

Writing the Mixed Methods Report

As illustrated in the boxed inserts in this chapter, findings from mixed methods studies can be presented in a number of ways. Many published studies do not adhere to the terminology of mixed methods, thus making it difficult to ascertain what design they used (see Box 3.3 for an example).

Assuming the two sides were kept intact, the findings are presented side by side, numerically, and thematically. Usually some attempt is made to interpret them in tandem and discuss the degree to which they converge or diverge. Gioia (2004), for example, provided a descriptive summary of her quantitative findings along with a presentation of the qualitative themes, and then ended with a graphic display showing how the two "sides" were related. If the mixing occurred earlier such that the data analyses followed one approach, the findings are usually presented in one format. Perhaps not surprisingly given the motivation to mix methods in the first place, researchers tend to favor the multiple findings option to give each side its due.

Challenges for Mixed Methods Studies

Carrying out mixed methods studies poses challenges of various and sundry kinds. Among the logistical hurdles, most researchers are trained in one or the other method (most often quantitative), but not both. Having dual competencies in a team effort can overcome this drawback, but the lone investigator is at a disadvantage. Mixed methods studies also require dual outlays of time and resources to ensure that both "sides"—quantitative and qualitative—are given sufficient attention to be rigorous (Stange, Miller, Crabtree, O'Connor, & Zyzanski, 1994).

Another logistical challenge accompanies oversight of the two sides when their rhythms and phases unfold in different ways. Qualitative data analyses, for example, start early in data collection and may result in going back out into the field for further sampling and data collection. Meanwhile, the quantitative side is proceeding in linear fashion, waiting out the data collection before beginning statistical analyses. The qualitative side, even though working with a smaller sample, takes considerable amounts of time and resources for transcription and data analysis not matched on the quantitative side. Given these tensions, the temptation to use a dominant–less dominant design is strong, and the quantitative side often comes out ahead in these situations.

Because mixed methods imply combining within the confines of a single study, questions can arise regarding when and where one study ends and another begins. In sequential designs, too much time elapsed may lead to the conclusion that two separate studies were conducted. In concurrent designs, the "sides" may have few or no interactions and integration is minimal, thus giving the appearance of two unrelated side-by-side studies.

There are also questions about the adequacy and provenance of the data. Are answers to a few open-ended questions on a questionnaire sufficient to be considered qualitative data? Will a scale or index administered during in-depth interviews yield meager descriptive statistics of limited value? Collecting qualitative data under heavily quantitative auspices raises serious doubts about its authenticity and richness (Morse, 2005). Moreover, qualitizing quantitative data is not the mirror image of quantitizing qualitative data (this sentence is an admitted mouthful). With the former, quantitative data are aggregated and clustered, and the resulting categories are based on decontextualized data that are hardly comparable to categories inductively derived from in-depth interviews or extensive observation. Similarly, a disservice is often done to deep and rich data when they are quantitized. Perhaps the best lesson to come from all this is that qualitizing and quantitizing should be done with great caution and transparency regarding the reasons for doing so.

The conundrum posed by triangulation also affects many a mixed methods study. When results from both sides are in accord, the researcher concludes (perhaps prematurely) that her findings are confirmed. As discussed in greater detail in Chapter 9, the meaning of triangulation has been expanded beyond corroboration to include completeness. Ethnographers, for example, often use quantitative and qualitative analyses for comprehensiveness rather than for validation. The problem arises over what to do when the qualitative and quantitative findings are neither convergent nor complementary. Some researchers present the two sets of findings, acknowledge the conflict, and ask the reader (and future researchers) to resolve the differences. Others use the discrepancy as an opportunity to inquire further, first to ensure that each of the "sides" is not flawed or biased in some way and then to examine and even use the discrepancy as an opportunity to broaden or revise the study.

Box 3.4 gives an example of a mixed methods study in which serendipitous findings from the qualitative "side" broadened the study and extended its impact to include new perspectives on barriers to breast cancer screening.

Box 3.4   Serendipitous Findings and Mixed Methods: An Example From the Harlem Mammogram Study

The Harlem Mammogram Study was a mixed method (QUAN+qual) study examining why African American women delay in responding to an abnormal mammogram (Kerner et al., 2003). Interviews included measures of health locus of control, fear of cancer, beliefs about racism, insurance status, and psychological distress. The less-dominant qualitative portion consisted of questions about their mammogram experiences and discussions of aging, racism, body image, and female sexuality. Data analyses were carried out separately by the quantitative and qualitative members of the team who had the requisite expertise. Both "sides" shared an interest in understanding delay (or timeliness) and maintained close contact as the analyses proceeded. The quantitative side used a multivariate logistic regression model to predict time to diagnostic resolution (within 3 months or longer). The qualitative side used a modified grounded theory approach to identify codes and themes. The qualitative data were intended to bring greater depth and understanding (a supplementary role), thus corresponding to "completeness" as a goal of triangulation. As it happened, they also contributed two serendipitous findings that would not have emerged otherwise. The first of these was the "air theory" of cancer which was subsequently noted in the literature (Freeman, 2004). This folk belief, which holds that opening the body surgically exposes it to air that can cause dormant cancer cells to grow and spread, was volunteered by several women during the qualitative interviews. Its relevance to our interest in delay was obvious because a surgical biopsy posed just such a threat. The second unexpected qualitative finding was about the physical and psychological toll of repeated diagnostic tests among women who had had multiple abnormal mammograms. A significant minority of women in the study had to undergo repeated and painful needle biopsies and other procedures (Padgett, Yedidia, Kerner, & Mandelblatt, 2001).The qualitative results were significant in ways that our multivariate model did not (and probably could not) take into account. How, after all, could we have anticipated or measured "air theory"? The results also turned out to have more grab than the statistical analyses that proved to be disappointingly thin. Contrary to our hypothesized expectations, the effects of income, insurance coverage, and systemic barriers were not found to be statistically significant. Among 30 predictor variables tested in the multivariate model, only the degree of mammogram abnormality and whether the patient was given information were significant (Kerner et al., 2003). Had we omitted the qualitative portion of the study, the underperforming quantitative model would have been the study's only finding for dissemination.

Mixed Methods Approaches to Program and Practice Evaluation

There are several ways that qualitative research can contribute to a mixed methods evaluation (Greene & Caracelli, 1997; Padgett, 2009b; Rallis & Rossman, 2003). Quantitative evaluations are good at establishing what works, but qualitative evaluations help to understand *how* a program succeeds or fails. Although admittedly more time-consuming, qualitative methods are less intrusive and less demanding than an experimental trial (Perreault, Pawliuk, Veilleux, & Rousseau, 2006). Qualitative researchers can fade into the woodwork and respond nimbly to the ebb and flow of organizational life. The addition of qualitative methods to a quantitative evaluation adds flexibility and depth (Drake et al., 1993).

Qualitative research is particularly well suited to *formative* and *process evaluation*. Hong and colleagues (2005) used ethnography to conduct a formative evaluation of an HIV prevention program with injection drug users. Their findings regarding miscommunications and cultural relevance were used to inform and improve the intervention that resulted. Program or treatment fidelity studies are also amenable to qualitative inquiry. The inner workings of many programs—the dynamic interplay of the actors, their differing perceptions of events, and the effects of culture and gender—are difficult to anticipate and measure. Indeed, there is no substitute for what can be learned from extended ethnographic observation of a program and its day-to-day operations (Felton, 2005).

Qualitative approaches also mesh well with social advocacy values in evaluation—they empower less powerful stakeholders (clients, lower-level staff, etc.) by giving their voices greater prominence in "finding the value" of the program. A mixed methods approach cannot guarantee a successful evaluation, but it is likely to enhance the depth and relevance of the findings.

Summary and Concluding Thoughts

The popularity of mixed methods is higher than ever before. Mixed methods approaches can bring unprecedented synergy, but they are not a panacea. A number of methodological and logistical challenges stand in the way of successfully integrating quantitative and qualitative approaches, not the least of which are the additional outlays of expertise, time, and resources needed to do justice to both "sides."

This chapter began with the archetypal possibilities based on sequencing and dominance. It also offered several examples of the complicated, even messy, mixed methods designs that characterize applications in real-world settings. The devil, as they say, is in the details. Determining what to mix from the qualitative and quantitative sides, when to mix them, and how to make the linkages takes careful advance planning. Not withstanding these challenges, mixed methods open the door to illuminating contrasts, whether done to corroborate, complement, or expand knowledge into new frontiers.

EXERCISES

1. The *Journal of Mixed Method Research* debuted in 2007 as a reflection of the burgeoning interest in method integration. Browse this journal (or another of your choice) and locate a mixed methods study of interest to you. Using the notational system from Table 3.1, how would you characterize the study's design?

2. In class discussion groups, take a look at Table 3.1. Which designs are most common and which are least likely to be used? Why?

3. Choose a public health program or practice of interest to you or your class discussion group and talk through how it could be evaluated using mixed methods. Choose a design from Table 3.1 and then specify how you would carry out the proposed evaluation. What types of quantitative and qualitative methods, techniques, or analyses would you use?

4. Think of a topic for which mixed methods would not be a good fit. Why is this so?

Additional Readings

Creswell, J. W., & Plano Clark, V. (2010). *Designing and conducting mixed methods research* (2nd ed.). Thousand Oaks, CA: Sage.

Greene, J. C., & Caracelli, V. J. (Eds.). (1997). *Advances in mixed-method evaluation: The challenges and benefits of integrating diverse paradigms.* San Francisco: Jossey-Bass.

Johnson, P. J., & Onwuegbuzie, J. A. (2004). Mixed methods research: A research paradigm whose time has come. *Educational Researcher, 33*(7), 14–26.

Miller, S. I., & Fredericks, M. (2006). Mixed-methods and evaluation research: Trends and issues. *Qualitative Health Research, 16,* 567–579.

Sandelowski, M. (2000). Combining qualitative and quantitative sampling, data collection, and analysis techniques in mixed methods studies. *Research in Nursing & Health, 23,* 246–255.

Tashakkori, A., & Teddlie, C. (Eds.). (2010). *The SAGE handbook of mixed methods in social and behavioral research* (2nd ed.). Thousand Oaks, CA: Sage.

Teddlie, C., & Tashakkori, A. (2009). *Foundations of mixed methods research.* Thousand Oaks, CA: Sage.

4

Getting Started

Study Design and Sampling

Qualitative research designs are flexible and iterative, but they also share with quantitative designs the need to be systematic, transparent, and as rigorous as possible. A qualitative design is systematic when it follows the methodological guidelines of a specific method or approach (e.g., a grounded theory study will unfold in distinctly different ways compared to a narrative analysis).

Qualitative studies are not intended to follow a predictable step-by-step format and thus offer the opportunity for creativity as well as the challenge of decision making on an ongoing basis. Miles and Huberman (1994) refer to the "second chance" (p. 38) afforded by the flexibility and groundedness of qualitative methods. Transparency entails keeping meticulous records of what is done and thus maintaining a degree of accountability for decisions made along the way. Although there is a lack of consensus on what constitutes rigor in qualitative methods, few would argue that adhering to some standards is not critical. (See Chapter 9 for further discussion.)

Some researchers begin with broad study questions that spring from intellectual curiosity, prior theoretical frameworks, personal experience, or a commitment to human betterment. Study questions are distinct from research questions or hypotheses in being more broadly conceptualized and not directly researchable as stated. An example of a study question might be, How do refugee families adjust to postwar resettlement? Research questions might include the following: How are family relationships affected by displacement? How are decisions made about returning or staying in the new location? Are there signs of resilience and strength that distinguish some families from others?

Reviewing the Literature

Study questions and research questions do not get formulated in a vacuum. Although more often assumed than articulated, the fund of knowledge brought to bear by the researcher can make the difference between an innovative study and a ho-hum or wasted effort. One's fund of knowledge may include personal and professional experience, but its quality ultimately depends on an extensive and ongoing review of the research literature. Thus, a researcher may be interested in studying intimate partner violence because she is an abuse survivor or has worked extensively with other survivors, but her study would be impoverished both conceptually and empirically if developed from these sources of information alone.

A systematic review of the literature—including relevant theories and research both quantitative and qualitative—prevents reinventing the wheel and producing a study with a resounding "what's new here?" from readers and audiences. Building upon previous work sets the stage for deeper description, conceptual development, and theoretical refinement. Not doing so runs a high risk of marginalization and irrelevance.

The length and organization of a literature review depend on the study's purpose. Dissertations have few if any restrictions on length and high expectations regarding comprehensiveness. In contrast, evaluation reports present background information in summary form. Public health research typically hews closer to the latter category and follows a focused and targeted review. Similar to quantitative studies, qualitative literature reviews are extended arguments, critically evaluating previous research and situating the proposed study as occupying an important niche in knowledge development. The literature review is also an arena for conceptual thinking and for applying the theoretical lenses that will be brought to bear.

What distinguishes a qualitative literature review is its lack of conceptual finitude. Conceptual and theoretical doors are left open wide enough to permit new ideas and serendipitous findings to emerge. Whereas the natural closure of a quantitative review is the presentation of hypotheses and their component independent and dependent variables, a qualitative review relies upon questions posed in an open-minded, curious manner.

Developing a Conceptual Framework

Literature reviews contain (and are often organized around) key concepts that are touchstones for the study and its research questions. A qualitative study's conceptual framework is not a contractual obligation. Rather, it is a guiding influence that ensures the study will transcend mere description (no matter how rich and compelling).

As discussed in Chapter 1, theories and concepts play an integral role in qualitative inquiry. This begs the question of how, when, and where this role gets played out. The various qualitative approaches answer this question somewhat differently, but all assume some reference to the world of ideas swirling around a particular topic. Conceptual frameworks are invoked in the literature review, applied during analysis, and revisited during the interpretation of the findings. The key is to prevent them from becoming overseers of the study.

Formulating Research Questions

Qualitative research questions are intellectually interesting and point the reader in the direction the study will go. Of course, the phrasing and intent of research questions vary with the study's approach. Take, for example, an interest in studying young women who are HIV positive and engaged in prostitution or other sex work. The following are some examples of research questions matched to the type of method.

> Ethnography: Are there tacit values, beliefs, and practices that characterize a local "culture" of prostitution? If so, how do these affect the women's decisions about personal health and HIV prevention? How do the women negotiate relationships with their clients and with fellow sex workers? What is daily life like for them?

> Grounded Theory: How do women with HIV balance sex work with other life demands? Are there common elements to their experiences that can be identified as part of a grounded theory of AIDS prevention among sex workers?

> Case Study/Life Course: What life events (childhood or recent) led the woman to sex work and to becoming HIV positive? How is her life story similar to or

different from that of other women like her? Does her life story reflect generational or cohort influences?

Phenomenology: What is the lived experience of being HIV positive? What is the lived experience of sex work? What are the essential elements of the lifeworlds of these women?

Narrative Analysis: What stories are embedded in their narratives? How do these women "voice" themselves and others in their social networks? What do these narratives reveal about exposure to HIV and AIDS prevention in sex work?

Action or Participatory Research: What are the needs of these women as they perceive them? How can researchers join with them in a partnership to conduct research that addresses these needs?

Any of these may incorporate theoretical and critical perspectives. For example, feminist researchers might include a focus on the constraints of gender roles in sex work and of sexism in AIDS treatment and prevention. What is least desirable are questions that resemble quantitative ones (e.g., "What are the barriers and incentives to seeking care for HIV?" or "Which services do women with HIV use?" etc.). Such questions yield thin, concrete responses.

Designing the Study

The word *design* sounds almost too orderly for the iterative process that unfolds in qualitative studies (Tesch, 1990). Most qualitative researchers opt for a straightforward description of what they plan to do and how they plan to do it, using as many descriptors as are applicable (case study, ethnography, phenomenology, etc.). The latter is necessitated by the fact that many studies incorporate different qualitative methods and techniques rather than hew closely to a single approach (Bryman, 2006).

Qualitative designs are distinguished by their recursiveness and flexibility, often weaving back and forth among research questions, data collection, and data analysis. In this fashion, the researcher may reformulate his research questions based on new findings, may seek new samples of respondents, or may pose new questions to existing study participants. Similarly, data analyses can precipitate the collection of additional data.

In quantitative designs, a formulaic approach puts the emphasis on minimizing external "noise" and threats to validity (i.e., "What you see is what you get"). In contrast, qualitative researchers pride themselves on viewing "noise" as an inevitable and even welcome part of naturalistic studies. Yet they must also convince their audience that they can (and will) produce credible, trustworthy findings. This means offering an explicit message of "here is what I/we plan to do," tempered by the conditional message that "these plans may be modified, but all analytic decisions will be justified and made transparent."

Questions Posed (and Needing Answers) by Qualitative Research Designs

Box 4.1 shows a series of questions typically posed by qualitative designs. Questions with relatively straightforward answers have them provided in parentheses. Questions without immediate answers are asterisked as "it depends." Perhaps not surprisingly, these questions cannot be answered without reference to the specific method being used as well as the scope of the study. Regardless, a qualitative research proposal should aim for as much specificity as possible. To be sure, overattention to detail may drain away the creativity that lends qualitative findings their strength and longevity. But creativity need not preclude planning ahead.

Box 4.1   Questions Posed by Qualitative Research Designs

"How many?" questions:

- How many study participants are needed?*
- How many interviews per participant? (Whenever possible, there should be at least two.)
- How many study sites are needed?*
- How many weeks, months, or years are needed to complete the study?*

"Should I?" questions:

- Pilot test the interview guide? (Yes!)
- Pay participant incentives? (Yes, if you can afford them.)

(Continued)

(Continued)

- Have comparison groups? (Only if your topic requires it.)
- Collect observational data if it is an interview-based study? (Yes—see Chapter 6.)
- Identify the strategies for rigor to be used? (Yes—see Chapter 9.)

"When?" questions:

- When should I start analyzing the data? (As early as possible.)
- When is there enough data to stop collection? (Usually at "saturation" point.)
- When should mentoring and supervision be sought? (Early and often.)

"How?" questions:

- How do I address ethical concerns? (More on this in Chapter 5.)
- How do I sample study participants? (Discussed later in this chapter.)
- How do I leave the field and end data collection? (See Chapter 8.)
- How do I analyze the data? (See Chapter 8.)
- How do I write and present the findings? (See Chapter 10.)

*It all depends.

The Element of Time

Flick (2004) notes the importance of time in design decisions. If concerned with temporal change, qualitative studies may be *retrospective* (e.g., life histories) or *prospective,* using longitudinal designs. When change is not the focus, qualitative studies may be "snapshots" (Flick, 2004, p. 148) or cross-sectional in design. Anthropologists, for example, talk about the "ethnographic present" as a compression of the lengthy period (usually a year or more) when they conducted their research in the field.

Prospective longitudinal designs entail multiple interviews conducted with study participants over several months (or even years). What makes a study "longitudinal" is the following: (1) its reliance on two or more waves of interviewing separated by a specified time interval, and (2) its ulterior motive of examining change over time. Iversen and Armstrong (2006), for example, conducted ethnographic interviews with low-income families over a 5-year period to portray their ongoing struggle with declining economic fortunes.

Specific Aspects of Qualitative Designs

Notwithstanding the looping back and forth that characterizes most qualitative designs, the description itself is fairly linear. Building on the questions posed in Box 4.1, the primary items to consider are as follows:

1. Which qualitative method(s) will be used? Include a rationale for this choice.

2. If the study is longitudinal, describe this, including procedures for retaining participants.

3. How many participants will there be, and how will they be sampled?

4. List the inclusion/exclusion criteria for eligibility.

5. How, where, and by whom will participants be recruited?

6. How will informed consent be obtained and human subjects protections maintained over the course of the study?

7. What types of data collection will be pursued?

8. How many interviews will be conducted per participant?

9. About how long will interviews last and where will they take place?

10. How (if at all) will incentives be paid and how much will they be?

11. How will data be managed and transformed, including transcription?

12. How will data be analyzed (including kind of software to be used)?

13. Which strategies for rigor will be used?

14. How will findings be presented and disseminated?

15. Give a timeline for completion of all study tasks.

Creating a timeline of tasks or a schema showing the study's stages is an excellent way of visually displaying what needs to be done and when, even if presented with a caveat regarding the flexibility that may accompany sampling or data collection. All descriptions should liberally cite the relevant experts in the literature and offer thorough descriptions and rationales.

One modest but essential way to enhance a qualitative study is to build in a pilot study. Little has been written about this in qualitative texts, in large part because of the unpredictable nature and frequent absence of fixed protocols in qualitative studies. In the NYSS, we conducted two to three pilot interviews and sought feedback on their content, sensitivity, and length from the respondents. This in no way foretold all of the complications that lay ahead, but it did result in an improved set of questions for the interviews.

Using Multiple Qualitative Methods at Different Levels

As discussed in Chapter 2, the topic of interest and scope of the study may lead to using more than one qualitative method and technique. It is helpful to distinguish between mixing at the method level (grounded theory, ethnography, etc.), at the level of data collection (focus groups, in-depth interviews, observation, etc.), and in use of analytic methods (coding, case study analysis, discourse analysis, etc.). A study of college drinking, for example, might pair ethnographic observation of local bars with case studies of selected clubs and fraternities where drinking is heaviest. (The amount of participation by the researcher, i.e., drinking beer with one's informants, should be monitored to ensure that field notes are accurate.)

Within a particular approach, it is not uncommon to use multiple types of data collection. Ethnography supplements its trademark participant observation with informant interviews. A grounded theory study might use interviews from focus groups as well as individuals. A life history study might go beyond first-person accounts to draw on participants' documents such as diaries, photographs, newspaper clippings, and so on. On the other hand, qualitative approaches such as narrative and phenomenological analyses do not lend themselves as easily to multiple data forms, given their almost exclusive reliance on interviews and narrative. A final note: Mixing may occur sequentially as well as concurrently, depending on the study design and scope.

Sampling Strategies

Qualitative researchers in public health sample a number of things, including places (clinics, neighborhoods, census tracts) and events (staff meetings, health fairs, religious festivals), as well as people. Sampling may begin with larger units such as health districts and then proceed to selected individuals at these locations (e.g., government officials, physicians, and community health workers).

Of course, the ultimate decision about whom to sample should be driven by the study's research questions and goals. As a general rule, qualitative researchers use *purposive sampling*—a deliberate process of selecting respondents based on their ability to provide the needed information. As Miles and Huberman (1994) note, qualitative sampling is done for conceptual and theoretical reasons, not to represent a larger universe.

Purposive sampling—also known as purposeful sampling—implies that a researcher interested in how cancer patients cope with pain will seek out respondents who have pain rather than randomly sample from an oncologist's patient roster. As such, it should not be confused with *convenience sampling*, that is, selecting respondents based solely on their availability. Convenience may lead a researcher to a particular site (e.g., a domestic violence shelter where she has volunteered in the past), but this should be done only if that site is most appropriate for the study. Patton (2002, pp. 232–242) describes various types of purposive sampling. Some of these are suited to the outset of a study and others are for later use. Initial sampling techniques are described here:

- *Extreme or deviant case sampling* looks for cases that illuminate the "outer edges" of a phenomenon, for example, obese children.
- *Intensity sampling* is similar to the above but the cases are not as unusual—children who are overweight, for example.
- *Maximum variation sampling* captures heterogeneity across the sample population (e.g., breast cancer survivors who had all types of adjuvant therapy [chemotherapy, radiation, etc.] as well as those who rejected such treatments in favor of alternative remedies).
- *Homogeneous sampling* is the opposite of the above, for example, narrowing the sample to include only those cancer survivors who rejected adjuvant therapies.
- *Typical case sampling* recruits "average" members of the population (e.g., teenage mothers with infants attending an urban pediatric clinic).
- *Critical case sampling* involves recruiting to illuminate the extremeness of a situation, for example, parents whose abuse resulted in the death of their child.
- *Criterion sampling* is selecting cases that exceed some criterion or norm (e.g., pregnant women whose body mass index indicates serious malnutrition). A variant of this, *nominations sampling*, asks knowledgeable persons to name or select eligible persons based on the study criteria.
- *Snowball sampling* entails recruiting one or more members of an isolated or hard-to-reach population and asking them to refer the researcher to other members of that group. In this way, a sample accrues, or "snowballs," as new referrals point the way to recruiting others. Examples include gang members, IV drug users, or members of a religious sect. A variant of this,

respondent-driven sampling (RDS) (Heckathorn, 1997), uses a sequential combination of snowball sampling with mathematical probability for selecting eligible referrals. RDS has proven to be a valuable means of addressing HIV risk among broad networks of IV drug users (Magnani, Sabin, Saidel, & Heckathorn, 2005).

Analysis-driven sampling techniques occurring later on in a study may include any of the initial sampling techniques previously mentioned, along with the following:

- *Theoretical sampling,* which occurs when inductively derived analytic concepts are used to guide the choice of additional participants. For example, a grounded theory study of recovery from drug addiction finds that individuals with spiritual beliefs appear more likely to manifest a "natural recovery" without formal treatment. Further sampling of individuals who have experienced "natural recovery" would explore whether they had also used formal treatment and the extent of their spiritual beliefs.
- *Confirming or disconfirming sampling,* which takes the logic of theoretical sampling a step further to seek out specific examples to test the validity of the grounded theory. An example could be looking for individuals who manifest natural recovery and spirituality without any formal treatment and (more importantly) those who do not. The latter, a variant of negative case analysis, ensures that qualitative findings are subjected to disconfirmation. Finding a "negative case" (e.g., a participant who naturally recovered but held no spiritual beliefs) may be the exception that either proves the rule or overturns it.

These categories offer the researcher much-needed terminology on specific sampling techniques. Not surprisingly, random sampling is a rarely used option in qualitative research. Aside from the fact that many study populations do not have a sampling frame from which to randomly select, the need for small but meaningful samples makes random selection techniques the least appropriate.

Sampling strategies should whenever possible identify inclusion and exclusion criteria to set boundaries on who is and is not eligible. Researchers must make special provisions if they seek to interview anyone who is under age 18 or a member of a vulnerable population (e.g., pregnant women, severely mentally disabled persons, and prisoners). Sharing the study's inclusion/exclusion criteria is essential for those helping to recruit for the study, for example, staff at a clinic who are asked to pass out flyers or otherwise help to identify eligible participants.

Two related observations are pertinent here. First, sampling strategies may change in response to study needs. One might, for example, start out with maximum variation sampling and then turn to a more targeted technique such as deviant case sampling. Second, the researcher should take steps early on to ensure that flexibility in sampling can be pursued and sampling goals attained. For example, one might anticipate the need for snowball sampling when studying a relatively isolated population. If recruitment is being carried out among certain types of clients or patients, it is advisable to obtain assurances (and evidence) of sufficient accrual from appropriate gatekeepers or else expand recruitment to more sites. Experienced researchers often have agonizing accounts of being promised a veritable flood of eligible study participants by an intake coordinator, only to be confronted with a trickle when the study began.

Sample Size Considerations

Different approaches have differing sample size considerations, and there are no hard-and-fast rules. Case study analyses tend to have small samples even for multiple case studies—a single case may suffice in some instances. Similarly, phenomenological studies aim for depth—sample sizes of 6 to 10 participants are common, but the numbers may be somewhat larger if resources permit. Grounded theory studies tend to have larger sample sizes, although still usually well short of a quantitative sample.

A few rules of thumb are helpful to remember: (1) the smaller the sample size, the more intense and deep are the data being collected; (2) larger sample sizes are needed for heterogeneity, smaller sizes for homogeneity; (3) sacrificing depth (length of interviews or number of interviews) for breadth (number of participants) should be avoided—if, for some reason, you are unable to conduct more than one interview with each study participant, a larger sample may be desirable; (4) larger numbers need not be shunned as long as the study has sufficient resources and honors rule of thumb #3. Given the flexibility inherent in qualitative sampling, a study may end up with fewer participants than anticipated (because the data became saturated earlier on), or it may end up with a larger sample because of the need to pursue new leads from the analyses.

Qualitative sample sizes taken out of context can be deceiving to the uninitiated. Hirsch, Higgins, Bentley, and Nathanson (2002) conducted an ethnographic interview study of 26 Mexican women to examine male sexual fidelity and risk of HIV exposure. At first glance, such a sample size would make most quantitative researchers cringe. But further reading on the study's methods reveals that each woman was interviewed six times—a total of 156 interviews. At the proposal stage, one needs to provide a projected sample size, but this should be accompanied by a caveat about the flexible nature of qualitative sampling to assure the reader that it is acceptable to end up with a sample size larger or smaller than anticipated. Because of a fundamental concern with quality over quantity, sampling is not done to maximize breadth or reach, but to become saturated with information about a specific topic.

Recruiting and Retaining Study Participants

Qualitative researchers go where respondents are and events occur rather than the other way around. These locations could be clinics, schools, churches, remote villages, homeless encampments, or any site where would-be study participants can be found. Gaining the cooperation of intermediaries such as gatekeepers is often critical.

Researchers in the helping professions are naturally drawn to studying the health or other problems of the populations they serve. However, this can be risky if they recruit study participants solely through treatment and service settings. Such a reliance excludes persons not in treatment and thus skews the sample toward the more severe or chronic cases or the highest service users. Of course, this may be the only way to access the population (or it may be the proper site given the study's goals), but intrepid researchers pursue alternative routes to recruitment such as advertising or snowball sampling.

Qualitative researchers use a variety of strategies for recruiting respondents. Human subjects committees are especially fond of advertising for volunteers because it is least likely to involve coercion. Cooperating sites and gatekeepers can help in distributing flyers or mailing introductory letters to potential participants. The researcher may make guest appearances at regular group meetings to describe the study and invite participation. At all times, he should have a script ready, either written or verbal, giving a brief description of what the study is about and what participation will entail. Attractive flyers with these points in bulleted form are the most efficient way to get the message out.

Obtaining the optimal sample takes careful planning and expenditures of effort. The wider one casts the net, the greater will be the need to screen in and screen out potential participants. Given the smaller sample sizes involved, it does not make sense to cast too wide a net and then create ill will by rejecting many would-be participants and disappointing gate-keepers and others who helped make it happen. The winnowing process, which involves rejecting some individuals who do not meet inclusion criteria and being rejected by others who do not wish to participate, can be time-consuming in such circumstances.

Retaining study participants is a key element of study success. High attrition rates in studies owe much to the lack of attention to techniques designed to keep participants engaged voluntarily (which is the only kind of engagement permitted). While essential for longitudinal studies, study retention also pertains to qualitative research because multiple interviews with each participant are optimal.

The relational aspects of qualitative research generally confer an advantage in this regard, but there are specific techniques that a conscientious researcher should consider using. These include asking for contact information, paying incentives, and offering a telephone number or e-mail address where participants may reach out with questions or concerns.

Researcher–Participant Dynamics: Gender, Ethnicity, Age, and Social Class

The dynamic interplay between researchers and their respondents—each affecting one another in not easily predictable ways—is a defining (and exciting) feature of qualitative inquiry. Feminist researchers have led the way in discussing this as a methodological issue (Fonow & Cook, 1991; Reinharz, 1992). Accepting rather than condemning its existence, they have explored how subjectivity shapes the study findings.

Although the researcher–respondent relationship can be influenced by many attributes, the most tangible are the "fit" (or lack thereof) in gender, ethnicity, age, and other demographic characteristics. Sometimes the researcher has little in common with her respondents. Elliot Liebow (1993) acknowledged stark differences in sex, age, race, and social class when he began his study of African American homeless women in Washington, D.C. Yet he was able to forge enduring relationships with the homeless women and write a moving portrayal of their lives.

A practical discussion of these factors and how they may be dealt with will be offered in Chapter 6. Perhaps it is sufficient to say here that gender and other disparities in the researcher–researched dyad deserve attention in the design of qualitative research, whether that attention is concerned with training and supervision of the interviewers, with ethical issues, or with how the findings will be safeguarded from bias.

Introducing the Three Main Types of Data Collection

Three types of data collection are dominant in qualitative research: observation, interviewing, and amassing documents. The latter is considered least intrusive or *reactive* (biased by the presence of the researcher). Secondary analysis of qualitative data is an option that is also low in reactivity, but can be problematic when earlier flaws are simply carried forward (Thorne, 1998). The variety of techniques nested within each of these broad formats will be the subject of Chapters 6 and 7. As shown in Box 4.2, the New York Services Study (NYSS) was large enough to encompass two types of research designs and purposive sampling techniques.

Box 4.2	Research Designs in the New York Services Study

The research designs for the NYSS indexed its specific aims. The study had two separate designs, the first based on life histories (collected in two interviews) and the second employing a prospective longitudinal mixed methods (qualitative-dominant) design. Sampling in Phase 1 used something rare in qualitative methods—a sampling frame from an earlier experimental study comparing enrollees in a "housing first" (experimental) program to those in "treatment first" (control) programs in New York City. We chose a type of purposive sampling (nominations sampling) in which the roster of earlier participants was independently scrutinized by two experienced interviewers from the earlier study and categorized as either "successes" or "non-successes" from the experimental and control groups. "Success" was a judgment based on mental functioning, substance dependence, and overall life functioning. Once the roster was divided into the four groups (based on consensus discussion), recruitment was initiated to ensure adequate representation from each group. The Phase 2 design required much more protocol development because it involved recruiting 80 clients from four city agencies, each of whom was interviewed three times over a 12-month period. In addition, each client's case manager was interviewed twice, once right after client entry and the second time after

6 months of program enrollment (or sooner if the client left the program). To enable tracking and retention, we planned monthly 10-minute check-in interviews with clients (for which they were paid $10). Recruitment of client participants depended on ongoing relationships with the referring agencies because intake managers were asked to follow our inclusion criteria and inform eligible clients about the study. (The $30 incentive smoothed the way considerably.) Tracking clients who left the programs was a challenge, with many relapsing and returning to the streets. The turnover in case managers required vigilance as well. Slippage in the best-intended protocols is not uncommon, especially with hard-to-reach populations. Compared to most qualitative studies (which are not longitudinal and multiphase), the NYSS was a large-scale effort.

Summary and Concluding Thoughts

Qualitative studies require careful thought to settle on the optimal design. Their contours are visible in a thorough review of the literature—theoretical and empirical. The literature review sets the stage with overarching study questions and specific research questions containing key ideas and concepts. The selection of qualitative approach(es), in turn, guides the design of the study and its implementation.

Like their quantitative counterparts, qualitative studies must address the element of time (longitudinal versus "snapshot" designs), choose a sampling strategy including the desired number of participants, develop ethical protocols for recruiting and retaining participants, and specify the number of interviews per person and the types of data to be collected. It must be clear if and when incentives are paid, how data will be stored and managed, what data analyses will be performed, and what strategies for rigor will be employed. Unlike their quantitative counterparts, qualitative designs are not linear (even if their description appears as such). Instead, qualitative designs adopt an iterative back-and-forth rhythm between data collection and analysis.

This chapter has posed numerous questions whose answers form the backbone of a study's planning stage. Although each approach has its own procedures, all share in common the need to transparently spell out what lies ahead to the fullest extent possible.

EXERCISES

1. Choose a topic of interest and formulate one research question suitable for each of the types of qualitative methods: ethnographic, grounded theory study, case study, and so forth.

2. Using either the same topic you chose from #1 or a new one, plan and write out your research design for one particular type of qualitative method. Include answers to the "how many" questions as well as which type of sampling strategy you will use.

3. Think of a "hard to reach" population and identify one or more sampling and recruitment techniques that would be most effective.

4. Imagine that you are applying for funding from a private foundation and a member of the selection committee says, "Your qualitative research looks interesting, but I honestly don't see how much can be learned from such a small sample." How would you respond to that comment?

Additional Readings

Corbin, J., & Strauss, A. (2008). *Basics of qualitative research* (3rd ed.). Thousand Oaks, CA: Sage.

Crabtree, B. F., & Miller, W. L. (1999). *Doing qualitative research* (2nd ed.). Thousand Oaks, CA: Sage.

Creswell, J. W. (2007). *Qualitative inquiry and research design* (2nd ed.). Thousand Oaks, CA: Sage.

Hesse-Biber, S., & Leavy, P. (2010). *The practice of qualitative research* (2nd ed.). Thousand Oaks, CA: Sage.

LeCompte, M. D., & Schensul, J. J. (2010). *Designing and conducting ethnographic research* (2nd ed.) (*Ethnographer's Toolkit*, Book 1). Walnut Creek, CA: AltaMira Press.

Marshall, C., & Rossman, G. B. (2010). *Designing qualitative research* (5th ed.). Thousand Oaks, CA: Sage.

Maxwell, J. A. (2004). *Qualitative research design: An interactive approach* (2nd ed.). Thousand Oaks, CA: Sage.

Patton, M. Q. (2002). *Qualitative research and evaluation methods* (3rd ed.). Thousand Oaks, CA: Sage.

Silverman, D. (2010). *Doing qualitative research* (3rd ed.). Thousand Oaks, CA: Sage.

5

Ethical Issues in Qualitative Research

The dynamic and ongoing nature of relationships in qualitative research raises a number of ethical questions (Christians, 2000; Punch, 1994). Some ethical issues can be anticipated and dealt with in advance; however, the flexibility of qualitative inquiry means that unforeseen dilemmas can arise at any time. As will be discussed later on in this chapter, ethical guidelines designed for quantitative research do not easily fit the exigencies of qualitative studies.

Deception and Disclosure

Deception (concealing the nature of the study and the investigator's role) is prohibited in virtually all research these days. The history of research deception, from Nazi medical experiments to the infamous Tuskegee study to Stanley Milgram's electric shock studies, makes its practice virtually indefensible. Of course, the harm incurred varies considerably—a high-risk medical experiment has far more potential for harm than an observational study of behavior in busy public spaces.

Three interrelated aspects of research deception are at issue in deciding whether it is defensible: (1) its necessity to carrying out the study, (2) its potential for harm, and (3) its intentionality. With regard to the first of these, human subjects committees have clear guidelines restricting use of deception to studies where the benefit outweighs the risk and the study could not be conducted otherwise. In these instances, researchers are required to put in place a number of safeguards such as debriefing subjects afterward.

The potential for harm is another variable. A number of landmark studies in the social sciences could not have been carried out without deception. LaPiere's (1934) study of racial and ethnic discrimination in the 1930s was based on his travels with a Chinese couple to various hotels and restaurants around the United States. The proprietors' discriminatory practices were, unbeknownst to them, contrasted with their previous survey responses stating they did not practice discrimination. If they had known the identity of LaPiere and his traveling companions, they likely would have behaved differently.

LaPiere's deception seems worth the risk, especially since harm was minimal or nonexistent given that no identities were revealed. Similarly, a researcher interested in unobtrusively observing panhandlers and pedestrians on a busy street can make a compelling argument for deception as having little potential for harm. To require informed consent would deny the naturalness on which the study depends because it would create serious distortion, or reactivity, in the behavior of those being observed.

Observational studies in public or semi-public places can be out of line if they involve reports of sensitive or stigmatized behavior. Laud Humphries' (1970) controversial study of gay men's behavior in public restrooms provoked cries of outrage when his deceptive tactics became known. Although Humphries countered that the study's findings justified the use of deception, few would defend his actions today.

If the legitimate reasons for intentional deception are few and must be carefully justified, what about unintentional deception? Human subjects committees would not countenance this on the face of things. However, in certain types of qualitative research (e.g., ethnography), it is virtually impossible to notify every individual who might cross the researcher's path. Consider a hypothetical study of staff–patient interactions in a rural health clinic. A good faith effort requires that any gatekeepers (e.g., the medical director) be notified in advance and that formal sit-down interviews occur only after gaining informed consent. Yet one cannot give advance notification to every individual passing through the clinic—every patient, concerned family member, and health worker—by telling them that they will be observed. Nor can one be expected to obtain formal consent every time an impromptu question is asked.

Promoting candor and transparency does not mean that participants have to be told every detail of the study or that every person within eyesight of the researcher requires full notification—not even the most stringent ethical guidelines require this.

Informed Consent

Because the vast majority of qualitative research involves active, face-to-face engagement, informed consent is an "ongoing and negotiated" process (Waldrop, 2004, p. 238). The basic elements of informed consent are these:

- A brief description of the study and its procedures as they involve participants (approximate number of interviews, duration of the study, etc.);
- Full identification of the researcher's identity and of the sponsoring organization (if any), including an address or telephone number for future contacts;
- An assurance that participation is voluntary and that the respondent has the right to withdraw at any time without penalty or loss of services;
- An assurance of strict confidentiality (which may be accompanied by two caveats: one regarding mandated reporting by licensed professionals as required by law and the other regarding the risk of a breach in confidentiality from other focus group members);
- Any risks or benefits associated with participation in the study. (Incentive payments are not considered benefits but, rather, reimbursement.)

It is also necessary to get explicit consent to audiotape interviews, along with assurances that participants may request that all or part of such recordings be withdrawn from the study. Most researchers bring two copies of the consent form (one for the researcher and one for the respondent to keep).

Special precautions are needed for studies involving members of vulnerable populations (e.g., pregnant women, prisoners, institutionalized mentally disabled people, and children). For studies of children and adolescents under age 18, written consent must be obtained from the parents and the child (children under age 12 may give verbal assent). For vulnerable populations such as the frail elderly, consent may need to be obtained from a guardian as well as from the respondent.

Signed consent may be waived under certain circumstances to protect the identities of vulnerable participants. A researcher studying gay and lesbian youth at a community center where they are considered emancipated would neither want nor need signed consent from their parents. The same would be true of undocumented immigrants who have reasonable fears that disclosing their identity would jeopardize their status.

The researcher should obtain the permission of gatekeepers whose approval is necessary to carry out the study, usually in the form of a signed letter. Such written permission is essential if their cooperation involves assistance in recruitment. *Gatekeepers* may include agency directors, clinic supervisors, hospital administrators, school principals, or the local health minister. To neglect this important task could cause delays and even imperil a study.

As discussed earlier, gaining informed consent for impromptu interviews during field observation is not plausible given their spontaneity and unplanned nature. In these instances, tacit consent is usually considered appropriate as long as the potential respondent is free to refuse to cooperate by simply walking away.

Obtaining formal consent has its drawbacks. Many researchers have commented on the off-putting effects of asking participants to absorb two or more pages of information cast in bureaucratic language and then put their signature on it. This problem is especially pronounced where literacy is low and understanding of Western research practices uncommon (Czymoniewicz-Klippel, Brijnath, & Crockett, 2010). The distancing and formality of the consent process have to be overcome to set the stage for the freer expression of an in-depth interview.

Coercion and "Deformed" Consent

The threat of coercion—whether heavy-handed or subtle—is a genuine concern in all research, especially in studies of vulnerable populations. Researchers tend to occupy higher-ranking social positions than their study participants and have institutional affiliations that can inspire feelings of coercion (not to mention real coercion). Thus, even carefully obtained consent can become "deformed" consent.

Human subjects committees have extensive guidelines to safeguard against coercion, including consent form language designed to assure prospective study participants that they are free to refuse participation and to withdraw from the study at any time without any loss of services to which they are otherwise entitled.

For practitioner researchers, the potential for coercion becomes problematic when the study involves patients, students, or coworkers who are familiar to them. For example, a health care administrator may want to conduct a study in her program or a teacher may ask his students to participate in his research project. Interrupting such a professional relationship to ask for consent can appear (and be) coercive even when handled sensitively. It is hard on the prospective respondents (who do not want to displease or who may fear retribution), and it can be hard on the researcher (who is trying to shift between research and work roles).

Confidentiality and Privacy

Qualitative researchers cannot offer the anonymity or safety in numbers that quantitative researchers can. They do, however, provide virtually ironclad guarantees of confidentiality. This means that every effort is made to ensure that the identities of participants are never revealed or linked to the information they provide without their permission. Breaches of confidentiality are undertaken only in dire circumstances in which there are serious risks of harm to self or others, particularly children. For licensed clinicians who are also researchers, mandated reporting may be a legal requirement and must be so stated on the consent form.

These precautionary measures represent a worst-case scenario that is extremely rare in qualitative research. Although they encourage candor and openness, qualitative researchers are not usually a sounding board for participants' thoughts of harming others (even when such thoughts exist). The same is not necessarily true of suicidal thoughts. In the NYSS, a few interviewees talked about suicidal ideation, usually as a thing of the past or in the context of help-seeking already undertaken. If a suicide attempt were probable and imminent, interviewers were trained to return to the topic after the recording had stopped, to ask if the participant felt he or she needed help, and to offer to make a referral to a hotline or other source of assistance.

Less urgent but still of concern are respondents' accounts of activities that are nonviolent but nonetheless illegal, for example, shoplifting, sex work, and drug dealing. Qualitative researchers cannot allow their personal or moral concerns about these behaviors to interfere with the promise of confidentiality. Intervening to prevent such activities would not likely be successful and in any case would end the research relationship (and possibly any chance of learning more about the respondents' risk-taking behavior).

Unlike quantitative research, a qualitative study runs a significant risk of breaching confidentiality in the reporting of results. Pseudonyms are typically used and inconsequential facts changed to help prevent this from happening; such breaches are less likely when the report relies on brief quotes or excerpts. More worrisome are vignettes or case studies in which individuals' life experiences are kept intact and their identities are traceable by others who know them. The more context and detail included in the report, the greater the risk. Gathering and storing visually recognizable images (photographs or video) of study participants runs a much higher risk of exposure of their identity (or at least a higher level of fear that this will happen). By comparison, audiotaping does not pose the same threat, since utterances are less identifying than visual images.

Sara Kahn, a doctoral student with whom I work, studied gay men who have successfully obtained asylum status in the United States due to persecution in their home countries. Their fear of being "outed" by descriptions and quotes in the study led to ongoing negotiations to ensure that no identifying information would be included in the dissertation or subsequent publications. These concerns are to be taken seriously. The men risk ostracism from neighbors and coworkers as well as reprisals from relatives or countrymen and -women living in the United States.

There is one other (albeit remote) risk of breaching the promise of confidentiality in qualitative research. Unlike attorneys and physicians, researchers do not enjoy legal protection from demands that they disclose information on illegal activities committed by study participants. Thus, an ethnographic study of drug dealers could catch the attention of a local district attorney and inspire her to subpoena field notes and transcripts. If a study's participants are deemed vulnerable to such scrutiny, the researcher may wish to obtain a Federal Certificate of Confidentiality (CoC) from the National Institutes of Health (available to all researchers regardless of funding source). The CoC gives legal protection to participants for a specified period of time. Thankfully, such dire outcomes are exceedingly rare. Prosecutors have better means (e.g., informants) to track down illegal activities and are usually reluctant to incur the wrath of local universities or research organizations.

Distress and Emotional Harm

Obtaining voluntary informed consent does not prevent one type of ethical problem from arising in qualitative research—the potential to cause emotional distress. Many qualitative interviews elicit intense discussions of painful life events such as sexual abuse, loss of a child, or a terminal illness diagnosis. Common sense dictates that such topics are not introduced gratuitously; they should be voluntarily brought up or, if necessary, inquired about carefully and empathically.

Although human subjects committees often assume that talking about sensitive topics is a recipe for psychological damage, emotional displays by respondents are not uncommon and are rarely cause for alarm (Seidman, 2006; Weiss, 1994). Rather than resent the qualitative researcher for eliciting such feelings, most participants remark that the interview is an emotional catharsis for them, a chance to express themselves before a nonjudgmental, sympathetic listener (Weiss, 1994).

The researcher should make advance arrangements for referrals to professional counseling if emotional responses are likely to occur. If a trained clinician, he should not provide this assistance directly (even if respondents request it). If offered, referrals should be made after the interview has ended to maintain the distinction between data gathering and the informal conversation that takes place when the recorder is turned off.

Incentives, Payback, and Maintaining Goodwill

Small monetary payments or other incentives encourage participation and partially compensate respondents for their time. As mentioned earlier, funded research projects routinely include incentive payments in their budget. The size of the payment depends on how much is being asked of the respondent in terms of time and inconvenience.

The decision regarding how much to pay respondents is ethical as well as financial. If one pays too little, the incentive value is lost. But if one pays too much (and especially if prospective respondents live in poverty), one risks taking advantage by purchasing their cooperation. Novice researchers usually consult with more experienced colleagues to find out the current rates of compensation for study participation. Payment of cash incentives may not be feasible for researchers who lack funding, especially students who are themselves struggling financially. Students I have known have offered inexpensive gift certificates to a coffee shop or grocery store, or persuaded a local vendor to donate small items (tote bags, sundries, deli sandwiches, etc.).

Another form of compensation or payback takes place naturalistically during the study. For example, a researcher who is spending time at a school interviewing staff might be able to offer an on-the-spot tutorial on a computer software program to help them with an administrative task. In the NYSS, a study participant recently released from the hospital revealed that he was intimidated by the subway system but needed to leave soon for a doctor's appointment. In the best possible response, the interviewer offered to accompany him to the subway to show him how to buy and use a MetroCard. Needless to say, payback has its limits—researchers should feel free to politely decline inappropriate requests such as going to a movie together, cashing or cosigning a check, hiding drug paraphernalia, and so on.

A final (and often overlooked) source of payback occurs after the study is completed—sharing the findings with the participants (Wolcott, 2009). Respondents often want (and deserve) to see the results of a study in which they played a key role, even if in the abbreviated form of an executive summary. In community-based participatory research (CPBR) projects, this is an essential component of the "contract."

Institutional Review Boards and Qualitative Research

A discussion of ethics in research would be incomplete without referring to government-instituted guidelines for adherence to standards of ethical conduct in the United States and many other countries. Such standards have their origins in the post–World War II Nuremberg Code and the 1964 Helsinki Declaration issued by the World Medical Association, both of which mandated that biomedical researchers obtain voluntary informed consent from human subjects. In the United States, a formal codification of these requirements in the early 1970s was prompted by revelations of the abuses of the Tuskegee Study. This study, carried out by the U.S. Public Health Service, was one in which syphilis was observed among southern African American men (and went untreated) for decades (Jones, 1993).

Box 5.1	Institutional Review Boards (IRBs) and Community-Based Participatory Research: An Uneasy Fit

As discussed in this chapter, qualitative researchers have their difficulties with IRB requirements since the latter are steeped in the protocols of biomedical research. This problem of "fit" is equally or more compelling with CBPR. Despite arising from a premise of sensitivity to human and community needs, CBPR is not immune to ethical concerns. Indeed, special problems can arise that are not common to other types of research (Flicker, Travers, Guta, McDonald, & Meagher, 2007). When researchers seek community partners, for example, they may unwittingly tap into and exacerbate schisms within the community. The same tensions can arise when making decisions about pay scales and incentive payments where monetary compensation might create divisions and competition for access to the compensation. Perhaps one of the more difficult problems attends decisions about a CBPR study's findings and ultimate dissemination. Researchers typically want and need to "stay true to the data" as well as their academic reward systems and thus publish findings even if they are unflattering to the community—an approach community members may oppose as harmful.

Flicker and colleagues (2007) examined application forms from 30 public health–related IRBs in the United States and Canada to see how well or poorly they fit with CBPR. Perhaps not surprisingly, there were numerous omissions or discrepancies linked to the IRB's ingrained emphasis on the risks and benefits of individual rather than community participation. For example, while 17 of 30 asked about financial conflicts of interest, only 3 IRBs inquired about potential imbalances of power between researchers and participants. None asked about equitable distribution of research budgets and resources characteristic of CBPR (Flicker et al., 2007). While retrofitting IRB protocols to fit CBPR would require substantial change, it would behoove IRBs dealing with community-based projects to be familiar with the particulars of this approach so as to ameliorate potential misunderstandings and mistakes.

Begun for all of the right reasons—egregious abuses of human rights in biomedical experiments—the formal guidelines promulgated under federal ruling 45 CFR 46 (the "Common Rule") in the United States have since raised a number of vexing issues. These include the wide latitude given to institutional review boards, shifting definitions of "research" and what thereby falls under their regulatory authority, and the methodological biases of these guidelines. The distance between what is prescribed by the federal Office for Human Research Protections (OHRP; www.hhs.gov/ohrp/) and the actual rules and restrictions implemented locally is a reflection of the interpretive freedom accorded IRBs. With over 6,000 IRBs located in hospitals, universities, foundations, and government agencies in the United States, it is no surprise that researchers encounter widely differing and at times seemingly arbitrary requirements (Bozeman, Slade, & Hirsch, 2009).

For qualitative researchers, a major concern lies in the lack of fit between the biomedical model implicit in IRB procedural oversight and the flexibility inherent in qualitative studies. Ethnographers in particular have been repeat offenders, or "IRB outlaws" (Katz, 2006).

The pervasive influence of the biomedical model shows up in a well-intentioned but intrusive paternalism that situates human beings as helpless "subjects." At the outset of the NYSS, we were required by the IRB to ascertain participants' capacity to give informed consent because they had a diagnosis of serious mental illness. We counter-argued (successfully) that an assumption of incapacitation, with the accompanying testing and implication of a guardian's consent, was itself a denial of study participants' free agency. Box 5.2 offers another example from the study.

Box 5.2   Misunderstanding What Qualitative Methods Are About: An Example

The bureaucratic "one size fits all" procedures of most IRBs set the stage for mis-understanding what qualitative research entails. In a recent study (following up on the NYSS), our team proposed conducting ethnographic site visits at two New York City agencies serving the homeless to observe staff interactions with clients and each other. In what was clearly applying protocols regarding partici-pants' right to have access to their own audiotapes or transcripts, our institu-tional IRB made its approval contingent upon permitting staff to have access to the ethnographic field notes. After conferring with medical anthropologist col-leagues on a listserv, we made a careful but firm reply to the IRB explaining that field notes are raw data capturing social interactions of a variety of actors. Even when no identifying information is included, the detailed descriptions of individ-uals might make them recognizable to their coworkers. Thus, to share these notes with a staff person would potentially breach the confidentiality of others. Fortunately, our appeal met with success when the IRB chair (a psychologist) conceded that field notes were not synonymous with interview transcripts.

Commentary: This lack of fit between IRB standards and qualitative methods can result in delays and undue burdens on the researcher. Over time, such prob-lems create a level of frustration and cynicism. However, early consultation, along with patient but firm responses, can resolve misunderstandings and lead to revised procedures that are more inclusive and less rigid.

Box 5.3	Protection of Human Subjects: Crossing National Borders

The Helsinki Declaration of 1964 prompted the Council of International Organizations for Medical Science (CIOMS) to put forth ethical guidelines in 1982, which were updated in 1993 and 2002. Beyond citing the need for voluntary informed consent, the CIOMS guidelines address the need for universal protections that are sensitive to multicultural settings and health systems, especially in developing countries. For their part, the World Health Organization (WHO) published "Operational Guidelines for Ethics Committees That Review Biomedical Research" in 2000. Similar to the CIOMS guidelines, the WHO document placed emphasis on the imbalance in power and potential for abuse inherent in Western research conducted in non-Western nations. This imbalance was revealed in the types of research being pursued as well as the ways in which such studies were carried out:

> The majority of biomedical research has been predominantly motivated by concern for the benefit of already privileged communities. This is reflected by the fact that the WHO (2000) estimates that 90% of the resources devoted to research and development on medical problems are applied to diseases causing less than 10% of the present global suffering. The establishment of international guidelines that assist in strengthening the capacity for the ethical review of biomedical research in all countries contributes to redressing this imbalance. (p. v)

As discussed in Box. 5.3, efforts to bring order to the patchwork of human subjects guidelines—with many nations having few or none at all—represent a step forward. Encouraging developing countries to have their own ethical governance procedures also helps ensure that the research taking place within their borders is responsive to local needs. Perhaps understandably, some developing countries' IRBs are charging fees upwards of $500, which can bring additional costs to a project. While international studies of researchers find little agreement on what guidelines should be uniformly enforced (Rivera, Borasky, Rice, Carayon, & Wong, 2007), a growing number of countries have adopted regulations governing protection of human subjects. As of 2010, a total of 96 nations have such regulations, according to the U.S. Office of Human Research Protections (www.hhs.gov/ohrp/international/intlcompilation/hspcompilation-v20101130.pdf).

Dealing With Moral Ambiguity and Risk

The moral ambiguity that surrounds naturalistic inquiry ensures that ethical dilemmas can arise at any time (Mitchell & Irvine, 2008). In-depth interviews can bring accounts of horrific or repulsive behaviors to the surface. Nora (not her real name), a participant in the NYSS, recounted being repeatedly raped by her biological father, who also verbally abused her during the assaults. Carlos, another study participant, told of being held over a stove's flame by his mother as punishment for childhood misbehavior.

Respondents may reveal aspects of themselves that cause shock, anger, and feelings of exasperation on the part of the interviewer. Nora ended her account to the NYSS interviewer by noting that she was planning to return to her childhood home to care for her elderly but still abusive father. Another NYSS participant boasted that he had fathered four children by two different women to "prove his manhood" despite having no income to support them.

Box 5.4   Moral Ambiguity in the Era of Online Social Media: One Graduate Student's Experience

Given the intensity of the relationship, study participants often want to befriend the qualitative researcher and the feeling may be mutual. Jennifer Mills, a PhD student I worked with, was studying young adult cancer survivors using in-person interviews followed by e-mail communications. Early on, several "friended" Jen on Facebook, i.e., asked her to join their personal online media site and thus have access to photos, messages to and from other Facebook friends, links to websites, and so forth. Young people are known to post online photos of intimate moments in their lives, and the lack of concern for privacy can be striking. "Friending" someone implies sharing such personal information and having mutual access to one another's Facebook page.

Jen's reply carried ethical and personal complications: She could agree to be their "friend" and have access to their online lives (with the potential for invasion of her privacy), or she could refuse and risk their alienation. Jen chose a prudent resolution: She e-mailed the participant and said she would agree to their request but was not comfortable reciprocating and allowing them access to her Facebook account (which was meant only for her family and friends). If they still wanted to give her access, she would be happy to oblige.

Commentary: This anecdote illustrates how unanticipated ethical quandaries can arise in qualitative research. Indeed, the above resolution opens the doors to new ethical questions regarding the potential "data" now being made available. A participant's blog or Facebook page is not unlike the diaries and photo albums of an earlier era, but gaining access to these requires getting specific permission.

The intensity and trust unique to qualitative research allows respondents to feel safe enough to utter despicable opinions or admit to illegal and morally reprehensible acts. The decision to intervene is rarely easy and frequently has unforeseen consequences. Steven J. Taylor (1987) wrote of an extremely difficult situation he encountered: physical and verbal abuse of developmentally disabled adults by the attendants in a residential facility where he was conducting fieldwork. Although appalling, the attendants' behavior triggered a moral dilemma for Taylor when he reviewed his options for responding.

Intervening with the attendants might have inhibited their abusive behavior (at least in Taylor's presence), but at a cost of breaching confidentiality and losing rapport (thereby ending his inhibiting presence and the study). Blowing the whistle and notifying the authorities (facility administrators, the police, or the media) was made complicated by the fact that facility administrators knew about the abuse, tolerated it, and even covered it up when confronted by family members. Taylor noted that pointing the finger at a few attendants was not likely to prevent future abuse because it was so prevalent and tolerated. Blowing the whistle also comes at a cost—breaching confidentiality and effectively ending the study.

Although acknowledging that there are occasions when intervening is worth it, Taylor ultimately decided to take no immediate action against specific individuals (thereby protecting confidentiality). Instead, he carefully documented his observations. After completing the study and writing about the prevalence of institutionalized abuse in treatment of those with developmental disabilities, he led a media campaign to expose the abuse and worked with legal advocacy groups to draw attention to its prevalence. What at first seemed morally unacceptable—continuing the study—gave him the commitment and knowledge to pursue these activities after the conclusion of the study (S. J. Taylor, 1987).

The primary issue for conscientious qualitative researchers caught up in such situations is not whether to do something, but what, how, and when to do it. The lesson of Taylor's experience is that initial impulses to take action should be weighed against foreseeable consequences. Put another way, the timing of taking action should be calibrated to fit the immediacy of the threat and the likelihood that such action will produce the desired result.

Moral ambiguity can happen in any study. Consider a few examples in addition to the one described in Box 5.4: A young woman with cervical dysplasia says that she will not seek treatment because she fears it will make her infertile. A gang member describes an upcoming initiation rite involving gang rape. An immigrant mother insists on finding a doctor to perform female circumcision on her infant daughter. The options for the researcher are the same as Taylor's: Do nothing, end the study relationship, intervene with the respondent, or blow the whistle to the authorities. Unfortunately, there are no clear-cut rules for which course of action to take and when to take it. Clearly, all of these strong emotions and raw experiences can take their toll on the researcher (Holland, 2007). In these instances, it is wise to practice bracketing (Ely et al., 1991), as described in Chapter 2. Traditionally associated with phenomenology, bracketing has been adapted more generally by qualitative researchers seeking to suspend assumptions, beliefs, and feelings in order to better understand the experience of respondents (Gearing, 2004). Debriefing is also important. In the NYSS, we scheduled weekly meetings to talk about the interviews, including their emotional impact. Interviewers and transcribers were also urged to voice any concerns individually.

Emotional stress is not the only risk a qualitative researcher may encounter. Although extremely rare, threats to physical safety may come from respondents, especially those with violent histories. Sexual come-ons and innuendo can also occur. Weiss (1994), for example, reported sexual overtures from his female interviewees. Such events can be discomfiting, especially when the interview takes place in the respondent's home or a private location where the researcher feels vulnerable. A rule of thumb in these situations is to plan ahead and to maintain professional poise, and to leave the premises if and when the discomfort level becomes intolerable. (See Box 5.5 for another example of ethical dilemmas encountered in a qualitative study.)

Box 5.5	Ethical Dilemmas With Multiple Gatekeepers: The Sonagachi HIV Project With Sex Workers in India

Cornish and Ghosh (2007) employed an ethnographic case study approach to describe the challenges of adapting to unequal and often exploitive social relations surrounding an HIV intervention among sex workers in a red light district in Kolkata, India. The Sonagachi Project used participatory methods in working with the women, but there were other more powerful groups whose cooperation was essential: the men's clubs who controlled the sex trade and the madams who employed the women. Not surprisingly, tensions were raised by the project's presence in the district, and its continuation was threatened several times.

To maintain its independence, the project's founders emphasized that they were not seeking to undermine the sex trade or to affiliate with any political party whose members benefitted from the trade. Indeed, the project had to compromise its pursuit of sex worker empowerment by including men's club representatives and madams on its governing committees and by acceding to their requests on occasion. Yet project staff also had their limits. On one occasion, for example, they felt compelled to intervene when a sex worker was beaten viciously and needed urgent medical attention.

Commentary: From the perspective of Western ethical standards, the Sonagachi Project adopted a morally reprehensible stance that not only sanctioned the existence of sex work, but also did not oppose oppression of the women by powerful exploiters. Instead, an ongoing series of delicate negotiations enabled the project to survive for over 14 years and realize many of its goals regarding HIV prevention and sex workers' empowerment. The tradeoffs that made this possible were a continual source of self-reflection and pragmatic decision making amidst enormous constraints.

Socially Responsible Research as Ethical Research

When it comes to social responsibility toward research participants, qualitative researchers have a distinct advantage because they are obliged to "go where the respondents are." However, for researchers committed to helping the communities they are studying, more is at stake (Pittaway, Bartolomei, & Hugman, 2010). When taking one's commitment to social responsibility to this level, the risks run higher in direct relation to the vulnerability of the community. Some problems can be anticipated, but others may happen despite one's best efforts. Consider the following hypothetical situations:

1. A public health team is conducting a needs assessment in a refugee resettlement camp in which there have been reports of alcohol abuse among adolescents living in the camp. Tribal leaders who act as gatekeepers have forbidden the team from asking about drug and alcohol use, but it emerges spontaneously during focus groups with the young people.

2. A public health researcher is working in a rural county in Liberia where she is designing and evaluating a health outreach program for new mothers. Due to cost cutting, she is told to use the volunteer CHWs (community health workers) affiliated with a regional clinic. Since a CHW has to be literate, all of the existing CHWs are men (as only males are permitted to go beyond elementary school in this rural area). The local midwives are upset and assert that the project further marginalizes women.

3. A team of environmental scientists has embarked upon a CBPR project with a rural community group concerned about contamination due to a lead mine nearby. Community partners are trained to work with the researchers in taking soil and water samples and interviewing residents living near the mine. The findings are jointly presented at a community forum. Attendees sharply disagree about what steps to take, and a rift opens between those who want to protest and get media attention and those who urge keeping a low profile since mining jobs could be in peril. The researchers are asked to take sides.

4. A group of AIDS outreach workers asked researchers at a local state university to help them design and evaluate a project that would promote safe sex and a needle exchange among IV drug users. Midway through the project, a state legislator and a religious group leader call a press conference to protest use of taxpayer funds for enabling illegal behaviors. The researchers are told to suspend their project by the university provost.

Each of these scenarios was not likely to be predicted in advance, yet its occurrence presents a threat to the survival of the study. Although the resolution of such ethical conundrums can be elusive, the more the researchers have a trusted relationship with the community, the more likely they will be able to forge a compromise that allows the study to go forward.

Socially responsible research also implies taking the larger structural context into consideration when interpreting and understanding the data. A study of persons with schizophrenia might, for example, conclude that they prefer to be isolated, if the focus is narrowly on what they say. Considerations of stigma and social exclusion bring an enlarged and more realistic perspective on their social isolation.

The incorporation of broader socioeconomic and cultural perspectives may seem to conflict with a focus on the intricate textures of people's lives seen from the inside (the emic perspective) rather than from the outside (the etic perspective). In fact, some qualitative approaches are less open to addressing structural issues—narrative and phenomenological analyses come to mind—whereas others such as critical theory and feminism are avowedly structural in focusing on inequality and its consequences. The majority of qualitative studies, however, occupy a middle ground in which the researcher may incorporate structural concerns at some (or all) stages of the study.

For a deeply disadvantaged population, it is not unusual (but nonetheless short-sighted) for researchers to interpret beliefs and behaviors as solely the product of personal irresponsibility or deficiency, even if that was the respondents' contention during the interviews. In the NYSS, we heard many stories of hardship that went far beyond having a mental illness diagnosis: life on the streets, joblessness, sexual and physical abuse, verbal abuse including racial epithets, and drug or alcohol addiction. Beyond noticing countervailing evidence (however tenuous) of individual resilience amidst all of this adversity, a deeper understanding of their situation cannot be had without reference to larger social and economic forces at work. These include drastic reductions in the availability of low-cost housing, cuts in social services, and the loss of unskilled and low-wage jobs. As well, there is ample evidence that childhood and adult traumas can have long-term deleterious effects. Last but not least, the powerful effects of antipsychotic drugs—extreme drowsiness, weight gain, involuntary muscle tics—can lead one to mistakenly conclude that drug abuse, poor personal habits, and apathy are in evidence.

Socially responsible research does not mean presenting a one-sided portrait that leaves out the less flattering aspects of respondents' lives. Qualitative researchers are not investigative reporters digging for dirt, but they are also not obliged to produce an uplifting portrayal devoid of nitty-gritty reality. This delicate balance between accuracy and sensitivity to respondents' needs affects studies of the despicable, the heroic, and the everyday people in between.

Summary and Concluding Thoughts

Ethical issues are omnipresent in qualitative inquiry. As with all research, qualitative studies must adhere to governmental guidelines ensuring voluntary informed consent; freedom from deception, coercion, or emotional harm; and protection of confidentiality and privacy. However, many gray areas remain when it comes to interpreting these guidelines and addressing ethical issues lying outside of IRB jurisdiction. Qualitative researchers frequently have the extra burden of educating their IRBs to ensure that the biomedical "one size fits all" model does not hinder their efforts.

The intensity and duration of the qualitative research relationship, in combination with its lack of strict neutrality, ensure that boundary maintenance requires constant vigilance. Notwithstanding good intentions, researchers who encounter morally ambiguous situations risk inappropriate responses such as giving in to the temptation to get too involved, showing disapproval of unsavory behavior, or letting their enthusiasm verge into coercion. The vast majority of qualitative studies pose a risk for harm no more severe than that encountered in everyday life. If properly observant of ethical guidelines, qualitative researchers can take comfort in the fact that their studies are likely to provide a satisfying and memorable experience for respondents.

EXERCISES

1. Go to the National Institutes of Health website (http://grants.nih.gov/grants/policy/hs/training.htm) or to your own institutional review board website and take the tutorial on human subjects protections. What are the basic elements of ethical research conduct?

2. Draft a sample consent form that includes the essential protections of human subjects for studying each of the following groups: (a) cancer patients in hospice care, (b) parents of children with autism, (c) adolescents aged 12–16 who smoke cigarettes.

3. Consider the possibility of conducting ethnographic research in a busy pediatric asthma clinic serving a poor inner-city population. How would you approach informed consent, being that you will be visiting for prolonged periods and at different times but cannot possibly request informed consent from everyone who will be visiting the clinic?

4. Consult the four "social responsibility" scenarios presented earlier in this chapter and discuss how each might be handled with the least harm done to the community.

Additional Readings

Christians, C. G. (2003). Ethics and politics in qualitative research. In N. K. Denzin & Y. S. Lincoln (Eds.), *The landscape of qualitative research: Theories and issues* (2nd ed., pp. 208–244). Thousand Oaks, CA: Sage.

Czymoniewicz-Klippel, M. T., Brijnath, B., & Crockett, B. (2010). Ethics and the promotion of inclusiveness within qualitative research: Case examples from Asia and the Pacific. *Qualitative Inquiry, 16,* 332–341.

Dickson-Swift, V., James, E. L., Kippen, S., & Liamputtong, P. (2006). Blurring boundaries in qualitative health research on sensitive topics. *Qualitative Health Research, 16,* 853–871.

Guillemin, M., & Gillam, L. (2004). Ethics, reflexivity, and "ethically important moments" in research. *Qualitative Inquiry, 10,* 261–280.

Holland, J. (2007). Emotions and research. *International Journal of Social Research Methodology, 10,* 195–209.

Katz, J. (2006). Ethical escape routes for underground anthropologists. *American Ethnologist, 33*(4), 499–506.

Malone, R. E., Yerger, V. E., McGruder, C., & Froelicher, E. (2006). "It's like Tuskegee in reverse": A case study of ethical tensions in institutional review board review of community-based participatory research. *American Journal of Public Health, 96,* 1914–1919.

Mauthner, M., Birch, M., Jessop J., & Miller, T. (Eds.). (2005). *Ethics in qualitative research.* London: Sage.

Mitchell, W., & Irvine, A. (2008). I'm okay, you're okay? Reflections on the well-being and ethical requirements of researchers and research participants in conducting qualitative fieldwork interviews. *International Journal of Qualitative Methods, 7,* 31–44.

Morse, J. M. (2007). Ethics in action: Ethical principles for doing qualitative research. *Qualitative Health Research, 17*(8), 1003–1005.

Pittaway, E., Bartolomei, L., & Hugman, R. (2010). Stop stealing our stories: The ethics of research with vulnerable groups. *Journal of Human Rights Practice, 2,* 229–251.

Rivera, R., & Borasky, D. (2009). *Research ethics training curriculum* (2nd ed.). Research Triangle Park, NC: Family Health International.

Thorne, S. (1998). Ethical and representational issues in qualitative secondary analysis. *Qualitative Health Research, 8*(4), 547–555.

6

Entering the Field and Conducting Observation

I n early ethnographies, the "field" was a faraway place where anthropologists went to spend a year or longer learning about the local culture. Nowadays, it can be a variety of places and situations, ranging from a finite location such as a clinic, school, or prison to a dispersed population such as transgender youths, persons living with hepatitis B, or methamphetamine abusers. What distinguishes being in or out of the "field" is the stage of the research vis-à-vis data collection.

Based on the premise that all qualitative research takes place within a "field" of action, this chapter will focus on observation as a form of data collection. Because gaining rapport is an essential ingredient for success, the early phases of reaching out to prospective study participants and sites are crucial. Success also depends on giving attention to the researcher's role as engagement with study participants intensifies.

On the Importance of Observation

Naturalistic observation, the hallmark of qualitative methods, has been relegated to a distant second place, with interviewing becoming the most prevalent qualitative method. This turn of events has its origins in the confluence of several interrelated factors. The first is the enthusiastic embrace of qualitative methods by professions such as teaching, nursing, and social work that rely heavily upon verbal communication. Second, talking and dialogue have intrinsic appeal due to their familiarity in everyday lives (P. Atkinson & Silverman, 1997)—the same cannot be said of participant observation. Finally, research interviewing has flourished as part of a larger phenomenon—the rise of an "interview society" in which television and radio talk shows (not to mention psychotherapy) feature "narratives of suffering" (P. Atkinson, 1997, p. 325) as the most authentic means of communicating the human experience.

The convergence of these three factors is not without consequences. Bemoaned as the "precariousness of a one-legged stool" (A. L. Hall & Rist, 1999, p. 291), interview-only qualitative research conveys the erroneous impression that anyone living in the "interview society" can do it—only good intentions are needed (Sandelowski, 2002). Beyond this naïve take on methodology are deeper concerns about the assumptive world in which interview-only studies take place. Thus, free-flowing narratives are considered to be superior because they give voice to study participants and provide a window into their "real" world. Such a realist assumption, more commonly associated with quantitative interviews, treats what participants say as having an inherent authenticity (P. Atkinson & Silverman, 1997; Sandelowski, 2002).

Taking everything said at face value is an error of commission as well as omission. Committing what Silverman calls an "Oprah Winfrey copout" (quoted in Gergen & Gergen, 2000, p. 1031), researchers dare not interpret what they are hearing, as this would dishonor participants. The pendulum appears to have swung from one extreme (the all-knowing researcher) to a romanticized other extreme (the all-knowing study participant). The error of omission comes from not considering the larger context of what is being said. In writing about his study of homeless booksellers in New York City, Duneier (1999) notes, "if I had simply taken the men's accounts at face value, I would have concluded that their lives and problems were wholly of their own making" (p. 343). Homeless men are hardly the sole architects of their fate, nor are they helpless victims of larger political and economic forces. Either of these two assumptions, taken alone, is obviously incomplete.

Is there a happy medium? To paraphrase a noted social scientist, "you can't generalize from the local, but you can't generalize without it" (Kotkin, 2002, p. B11). Readers of qualitative research are asked to trust the authors as guides leading them into new understanding, but researchers must earn this trust. To do so, we provide sufficient detail to assure readers of our immersion in the setting and data, but we are also obliged to make connections "up and out" to the larger context of opportunities and constraints. The reader may be asked to take a "leap of faith" (Duneier, 1999, p. 343) in this regard, but the leap should have a credible landing.

Here is where interview-only (as opposed to interview-intensive) research is problematic. Confining a study to interview data deprives it of the broader interpretive power that comes from observation (Agar & McDonald, 1995). An interview-intensive qualitative study can benefit from systematic and recorded observations of the interview context (the setting, nonverbal communication, etc.). Beyond the immediate surroundings of the interview lie opportunities to shadow participants and enter their worlds naturalistically—admittedly not always possible but at least worth considering (Kusenbach, 2003; McDonald, 2005).

Without a doubt, interviews will continue to be the staple of qualitative research—talking and listening are deeply woven into the fabric of our being. This chapter represents an attempt to swing the pendulum back a bit by emphasizing observation. We begin with preparations for entering the field.

Getting Permission(s) and Announcing the Study

After spending a considerable amount of time conceptualizing and designing the qualitative study, the cerebral gives way to the social. For most researchers, this is energizing, the time when all of the planning finally gets put to the test. Qualitative studies may be site-specific, person-centered, or both. Either way, it is common for a study to have some sort of institution and other authority involved. Here are a few examples from public health students with whom I have worked.

- Gregory was involved in a hypertension control project in a Filipino immigrant community made possible by his relationship with community leaders.
- Laura conducted a study of home and hospital births in Liberia that required cooperation from hospital administrators, doctors, and midwives.

- Nicholas worked on an oral health needs assessment on an American Indian reservation and obtained permission from tribal authorities.
- Miriam engaged in community-based participatory research with a group of "canners," or homeless persons who earn money by recycling discarded bottles and cans. She was able to gain entrée through volunteering with the group and working closely with the group's leadership.

Gaining entrée requires differing degrees of outreach and engagement ranging from placing an Internet notice or posting flyers to protracted negotiations including additional reviews by institutional review boards at various study sites. It is best not to take anything for granted. An administrator, agency, or community may have been friendly in the past and then bristle at the prospect of being put under scrutiny in the name of research. Similarly, study participants and communities often have legitimate concerns about the potential for human subjects abuse or negative portrayals (Malone, Yerger, McGruder, & Froelicher, 2006). Qualitative researchers have to accept the fact that the word *research* may conjure images of "human guinea pig experiments" and exploitation. (The use of the label *subjects* reinforces this image.) Substitution of terms such as *research project* or *study participant* is less distancing and more consonant with the realities of a qualitative study.

Finding the gatekeeper(s) and getting permission is an essential first step. In approaching such individuals, the researcher should be direct and forthright about the study's overall goals and the human subjects protections being offered. The study's benefits should not be overstated, nor should its risks be understated. It is also important to inform gatekeepers and others about the time-consuming and involved nature of qualitative research. If an incentive or other reimbursement is being offered, it should not be used as leverage or coercion.

It helps to anticipate gatekeepers' concerns or questions. In the NYSS, program directors expressed doubts about paying cash incentives, worried that study participants would spend the money on drugs and alcohol. Although we were prepared to substitute movie tickets or subway MetroCards as a last resort, our counterargument that study participants deserved the same choices as other adults was eventually accepted.

"Announcing the study" refers to laying the groundwork for observation or interviewing that is specific to a site. As with the usual procedures of informed consent, this involves full disclosure of one's identity, the purpose(s) of the study, its voluntary nature, and the protection afforded by strict confidentiality. If field notes will be taken, this must also be stated so that everyone knows that they might be observed. Other expectations of cooperation, such as help in recruiting, participation by staff in focus groups, and so on, must be clearly specified. For a clinic or agency, this can usually be handled by attending staff meetings to explain the study and answer questions. For larger entities such as multisite programs or health districts, letters of approval by gatekeepers can be sent to local authorities to smooth the way. Studies of neighborhoods often depend on cultivating the goodwill of civic leaders, clergy, and similar authority figures.

Observational studies bring special considerations. With the exception of research sites located in busy and open public spaces, the researcher should broadcast information about the study as widely as possible. During intensive participant observation, the researcher's prolonged presence gives ample opportunities for such self-identification. For sporadic or less intense involvement, having flyers and gatekeeper permissions handy and being available for questions goes a long way toward allaying suspicions. Of course, any contacts that lead to formal interviewing will trigger the need for informed consent.

If a site is being asked to provide assistance with multiple tasks over a period of time, a *memorandum of understanding* (MOU) is helpful at the outset to specify responsibilities of the respective parties. MOUs can be a reference point for everyone to clarify roles and reduce misunderstandings. A simple one-page bulleted list of responsibilities for the site and the researcher is a good start. Of course, an MOU should not lock the research in too stringently, because protocols need to remain flexible.

All of this interaction can produce a difficult situation if researchers find themselves too closely identified with gatekeepers whom participants view with suspicion or distrust. Potential participants can also get confused when well-meaning but overly enthusiastic gatekeepers assist in study recruitment. Of course, not all qualitative studies have to seek permission from formal gatekeepers (e.g., those soliciting volunteers through advertising or informal networks).

Obtaining and Maintaining Rapport

Once all formal permissions have been obtained, what James Spradley (1979) refers to as the "rapport process" (p. 78) takes center stage and continues until the study is over. Rapport can begin on a number of levels, depending on the complexity and length of the study. At a minimum, *rapport* refers to the sense of respect, trust, and positive regard between researcher and study participants that enhances openness in information sharing. Rapport also refers to maintaining good relations with study sites and their representatives. Paying participant incentives facilitates the development of rapport but can never substitute for interpersonal skills.

Spradley (1979) cautions that the mutual enjoyment typical of study participation does not necessarily translate into deep friendship or affection. A researcher and study participant do not have to like one another to have rapport. The first encounter, often awkward, should set the stage for future exchanges. Once a participant is engaged in the study, rapport is maintained or deepened by careful attention to changes that might signal distraction or fatigue. It is also enhanced by engaging in small talk before and after the interview (with the tape recorder turned off) as well as by the psychological benefits of the interview itself.

Presentation of Self in the Field

Qualitative researchers vary in how they present themselves, depending on their personal preferences as well as the particular setting being entered. Erving Goffman (1961), for example, adopted a marginal stance, detaching himself as he observed asylums and other institutions. At the other end of the continuum, feminist researchers advocate a research partnership in which roles are blurred and researchers are actively engaged in coproducing findings with respondents (Reinharz, 1992). Most qualitative researchers present a "self" somewhere in between that of a marginal outsider and an intimate insider.

The researcher is obliged to enter the field "with an open mind, not an empty head" (Fetterman, 1989, p. 11). In other words, the researcher should be knowledgeable enough about the topic to prevent unnecessary interruptions that disrupt the flow of the interview. In the NYSS, interviewers were trained to be familiar with the slang words for drugs (e.g., crack cocaine is "rock," marijuana is smoked in "blunts," and "benzos" are anxiety medications abused on the streets). Similarly, the terms "SSI" (supplemental security income) and "rep payee" were common parlance in interviews. These shorthand references to federal disability income and representative payee status can be mentioned by the study participant without having to explain to the interviewer what they mean. This leaves time for explorations with more depth and nuance, for example, questions about what it means to have SSI as a steady source of income or to have someone else in control of one's finances.

The interviewer's mode of dress and demeanor also deserves attention. Because dressing up can appear elitist or patronizing and dressing down can come off as disrespectful, dressing in a casual and neat manner usually works the best. Demeanor is a bit trickier because it involves one's personal style of communication and engagement with others. The researcher's creativity and intellectual curiosity should not be squelched; qualitative interviews usually rise above the mundane when the researcher is enthusiastic. However, when a researcher expresses too much individuality, it can detract from the real experts (the study participants). Optimally, the researcher is empathic and understanding without sacrificing professionalism. Maintaining a sense of humor, a willingness to be wrong (a lot), and an eagerness to learn is a winning combination.

Issues of Identity: Gender, Age, Race/Ethnicity, and Social Class

Whereas mutable characteristics such as dress and demeanor can be adjusted, relatively fixed traits such as sex, age, race/ethnicity, and social class must also be considered. Socially constructed meanings associated with gender, race, and class identity often come into sharp focus in qualitative research relationships and can become more complicated when the researchers and participants come from different cultural backgrounds. There are potential advantages as well as disadvantages to this situation. In her study of psychiatric outpatients living in the community, Sue Estroff (1981) made these observations:

> Being female helped and hurt. Over half of the subjects were men. My gender served as an entree to contacting them and eliciting some interest, but it created tensions as well. Many had never had a female friend, that is, a symmetrical, platonic, heterosexual relationship. This led to some confusion on their part when their sexual advances offended me, and to reluctance on my part in entering situations . . . which might be misconstrued. (p. xvii)

A relationship of mutual respect need not be based on sameness; the ultimate success of the study depends primarily on the skills of the researcher (Manderson, Bennett, & Andajani-Sutjaho, 2006). In addition to their demographic traits, researchers carry a number of identities into the field that they have acquired over time. These identities can be professional (student, professor, practitioner), personal (partner, parent, sibling), political (feminist, antiwar activist, animal rights advocate), and recreational (soccer fan, pianist, marathon runner). How, if at all, these identities influence the study is largely a matter of context and appropriateness.

Researcher Self-Disclosure: How Much Is Enough? How Much Is Too Much?

There are no prohibitions on personal disclosure in qualitative inquiry; some is to be expected as part of the give-and-take required to maintain rapport and trust. The overriding questions are these: Which "selves" should the researcher reveal? When is it appropriate to do this? Are there dangers to such revelations?

Qualitative researchers generally adhere to the advice to be "truthful but vague" (S. J. Taylor & Bogdan, 1984). One should never lie if asked a question, but should use considerable discretion in how much to reveal. Weiss (1994) suggests providing the basic "business card" information, but others assert that sharing personal information encourages fuller disclosure by respondents and promotes greater equality (Gair, 2002; Reinharz, 1992).

Interviewees often parry with questions of their own that require on-the-spot decisions on whether and how to respond. Take the hypothetical example of a graduate student–researcher who is a social worker, a parent, a cancer survivor, and an avid fan of heavy metal music. She is obliged to reveal her status as a student right away because this is the requisite "self" conducting the study. If the study involves potentially harmful subject matter, she will also have a caveat in the consent form regarding her legal status as a mandated reporter of child or elder abuse. Whether she has the occasion to reveal her musical tastes or status as a cancer survivor and parent depends on the context.

A researcher's disclosure of his various selves and life experiences cannot follow a strict protocol but is usually better confined to the before-and-after chat that accompanies each interview. During the interview, such decisions should take into account a risk–benefit equation balancing rapport with the potential for bias or intrusiveness. It can be entirely appropriate for the researcher to identify himself as being a military veteran or a recovering addict, but this should not be done gratuitously or appear as attention-seeking behavior.

Observation in Qualitative Studies

Imagine trying to fully understand how a hospice, refugee camp, or psychiatric ward operates by relying solely on verbal description. First of all, those who have more to hide usually hide it more. Second, many individuals are either unaware of goings-on in their midst or have spotty recall. As discussed in the previous chapter, the days of deception in observation are largely over. With rare exceptions, qualitative researchers develop and follow observational protocols that involve full disclosure.

It is helpful to distinguish between observation as a mode of qualitative data collection and *participant observation*, the centerpiece of ethnographic fieldwork (Emerson, 2001). While the latter assumes the primacy of immersion and interaction within a specific environment, the former is less site-specific and often used in conjunction with interviewing (thus being less intense and time-consuming). Although the dividing line between these is often blurry, we will focus more on the former with varying amounts of participation accompanying the observation.

Even minimal amounts of participation require careful consideration given the potential for *reactivity* (changes due to the researcher's presence). Think of a continuum ranging from full participation (living with the study population for a prolonged period and carrying out daily activities much as they do) to unobtrusive observation with little or no interaction. The risks at the high-involvement end of the continuum include researcher fatigue and some version of "going native" (losing sight of the researcher role). At the low level of involvement, avoiding interaction means foregoing a valuable means of learning in situ.

Both extremes are more difficult to accomplish compared to mid-level participation that is selective and contextual. If the study is site-centered, attendance at carefully sampled events—staff meetings, street festivals, political protests, support group meetings, and so on—can be extremely useful in documenting the range of activities. If the study is largely person-centered, getting permission to shadow study participants on their daily rounds of activities or on selected outings gives added value to what is otherwise entirely dependent on the participants' verbal accounts (Kusenbach, 2003). Sampling of events may be representative (e.g., varying by time of day, types of participants) or purposive (e.g., attending clinic days reserved for new mothers or shadowing a study participant who is a community health worker.

Some qualitative methods do not draw on observational data, for example, those relying on historical documents or narrative and other textual analyses. Some behaviors are too intensely private or risky to observe, for example, unsafe sex, self-mutilation, and IV drug use come to mind. Leaving aside these exceptions, it is safe to say that most qualitative studies benefit from collecting observational data, even those that are interview-intensive.

"Doing" Observation: The Best (and Only True) Way to Learn

Despite volumes of "field wisdom" passed on by ethnographers (Sanjek, 1990), the demands of qualitative observation can only be appreciated with hands-on experience. Public health students in my qualitative field methods course react similarly during their first participant-observation assignment—an initial response of "what a refreshing break from the usual class assignments" gives way to reality after an hour or two spent in the field. Post-hoc comments run along these lines: "I couldn't decide what to write down"; "There was so much going on, I didn't know where to start"; and "I've never felt so self-conscious before."

We are all participant observers in a way—nothing less is required when entering an unfamiliar situation, whether it is the latest nightclub or a coveted job interview. Yet qualitative research demands a more systematic, thorough, and nonjudgmental form of observation than the necessarily self-interested and selective observations one makes in daily life.

According to experts in ethnographic techniques (Agar, 1980; LeCompte & Schensul, 2010; Spradley, 1979), the best approach is to begin by casting a wide net and then move to more focused observation as the study's aims and major themes begin to crystallize. All of the senses are involved—sounds and smells can convey important meaning and context. Ethnographers usually seek out one or more *key informants* (knowledgeable individuals who can supply valuable information). Although the term *informant* is a regrettable holdover from earlier days, it connotes what is being sought because the individual is not asked to talk about personal experiences.

To illustrate the unique powers of observation with all of the senses, consider a typical homeless men's shelter. In photographs, it can appear relatively benign, for example, rows of beds with men sitting or lying on them. But a few visits for field observation will bring the sensory experience of the shelter to full life. Pervasive theft, drug use, and physical intimidation are the norms of life in the public shelter system, as recounted by residents and often barely concealed from visitors. The sensory stimuli add an extra dimension or two. The smells—body odor (few working showers), poor sanitation (nonfunctioning toilets), greasy cooking, and powerful chemical disinfectants—can be overpowering. However, the noise and lack of privacy are often the most disturbing aspects of shelter life—the cacophony of sounds from dozens (or hundreds) of men crowded into close quarters, cursing and shouting (including from guards and staff), some in the throes of drug-induced or mental psychoses. Usually required to leave the premises for the day, weary occupants return at night for rest, but get little. Residents' accounts of municipal shelter life are often dismissed as exaggerated or a flimsy cover for preferring the freedom of the streets. But researchers' firsthand observation more often than not validates these portrayals of homeless shelters as multisensory hazards to health and well-being.

Public health students carrying out observation exercises can provide vivid accounts based upon multiple stimuli, whether visual (rats, trash, polluted streams), aural (urban noise), or olfactory (rotting garbage, tobacco smoke, raw sewage). Indeed, many public health problems are detectable through the senses and in vivo. As discussed later in this chapter (Box 6.3), such clues can supply critical information in addition to interviews.

Recording Observational Data

Observation protocols . . . cannot be treated as faithful reproductions or unproblematic summaries of what is experienced, but should be seen, rather, for what they are: texts written by authors, using their available linguistic resources, to give a meaningful summary of their observations and recollections after the event. (Luders, 2004, p. 228)

Field notes are the necessary if imperfect representation of what is experienced during observation (Emerson, Fretz, & Shaw, 1995). Their quality is improved significantly by adhering to two practices. First, field notes should be taken either in real time or very soon thereafter because memory erodes dramatically within the first 24 hours after an event. Second, it is important to avoid the clouding or distorting effects of "filters," whether personal predilections or theoretical allegiances (see Box 6.1). No observer is a bias-free instrument, but attending to this fact is the requisite first step.

Much has been written addressing the "why, what, and how" questions of field note taking. Answering "why" is the easiest to do: Logging one's observations produces valuable raw data that can lead to more focused follow-up via interviewing or additional observation. The "what" of field note taking depends on the topic of interest, as no one can presume to record everything. General suggestions regarding what to look for in the initial phase include physical space, actors, behaviors, interactions, relationships, and affect (expressions of feelings or emotions; Lofland & Lofland, 1995). If one is observing a bounded physical space, it is useful to draw a map or floor plan to add a spatial dimension to understanding what is happening. An agency where staff share cramped cubicles will have a different feel from one where private work space is the norm.

The "how" of field note taking requires a good deal of flexibility, sensitivity to the situation, and practice. It is easier to take notes (or speak into a recorder) in busy public spaces where one can remain relatively inconspicuous. But there are many occasions when writing notes would intrude on the natural course of events and even provide cause for offense. For these occasions, Lofland and Lofland (1995) describe a sequence of taking mental notes—committing to memory as much as possible—followed by brief jottings or speaking into a tape recorder. (Retreating to the bathroom is a favorite technique for accomplishing this.) At the end of the day, one can write in greater detail.

Lofland and Lofland (1995, pp. 89–90) provide a number of helpful hints for field note taking:

1. Aim for the concrete and specific in describing behaviors and events. At the beginning, try to avoid any inferences, whether your own or volunteered by others.

2. Try to distinguish between the different types or levels of observational data based on their proximity to the event being observed (see Box 6.1 for an example). First-order data such as verbatim accounts are recorded either during or immediately after the period of observation. The second level of data involves paraphrasing conversations and less certain recall after observation has taken place. Ideas regarding new directions and inferences are further along the continuum of removal from the event and are periodically recorded in analytic memos. The final level of abstraction, concept development and theory generation, involves generating a meaningful explanatory framework that has been developed from the ground level up.

3. Record observations of yourself—your impressions, feelings, and concerns. You can bracket this information in your field notes or log it separately in a diary. Keeping a running commentary of personal reactions and feelings serves two related purposes. First, it is an outlet—a

place to unload the inevitably human reactions to prolonged contact with others. Second, it provides a means of identifying personal biases and devising ways to manage them.

4. Strive for balance—don't let yourself become lost in a forest of minutiae, yet don't lose the tendency for compulsiveness that motivates the best field observers. Even small amounts of time spent in the field translate into lengthy notes. The ratio is around 6 to 1—6 hours of recording for every hour of observation.

Box 6.1	The Distinction Between Observation and Interpretation (moving from data collection to analysis)

Raw description in field notes is balanced with (and distinct from) reasonably grounded inferences and higher-order interpretations (the latter requiring multiple sources of data to "work"). Of course, these distinctions are not always clear. Examples below are from a hypothetical study of secondhand smoke exposure on a college campus. Good examples are in italics and bad ones in regular font. Can you appreciate the differences as well as the similarities?

1. **Raw description:**

   Good: *I observed 10 casually dressed young people standing around under the portico entrance to the library, 8 of whom were standing alone and smoking (6 male, 2 female). The other two people (a man and a woman) were older, well-dressed, and engaged in a spirited conversation. A nearby planter contained numerous cigarette butts and the smell of cigarette smoke was strong. Some people entering the library waved their hands in the air as they passed through, but the smokers showed no reaction. In contrast, there were three people standing outside of the student center across the street and none of them was smoking.*

   Bad: There were several students standing around smoking and looking bored plus there was an older married couple arguing nearby. Across the street were more students talking but not smoking.

2. **Inference from above description:**

   Good: *Second-hand smoke is a problem at the library entrance more than at other campus buildings. Moreover, the portico design contains the smoke*

   (Continued)

(Continued)

and makes its effects concentrated. It is likely that this covered entrance is more attractive for smokers since it protects them from the elements. Males are more likely to do this than females. Those entering the library show their displeasure by waving their hands to dispel the smoke, but this does not deter the smokers.

Bad: The library attracts smokers to use its services and the other campus buildings do not. Male students like to hang around outside, but female students and older people do not.

3. **Interpretations/hunches/hypotheses (which would need further testing via additional data):**

Good: *Heavy smoking is associated with students "taking breaks" during studying, i.e., could it be a stress-reducer? Preliminary hypotheses and public health implication: Would prohibiting smoking within 20 feet of the building prevent this problem? Or would it only "push" smokers to another location? Would a harm-reduction approach work, e.g., providing a special room for smokers in the library? If stress of studying is part of the reason for smoking, would stress-reduction classes in the library be a good move?*

Bad: Gender is a determinant of smoking behavior on campuses. Smoking has been linked to stress and anxiety; therefore, male students are more stressed than female students.

1. **Personal reflections (There is no good or bad!):** *I was disgusted by the smokers' indifference to others. This university should be more aggressive in its prohibitions OR I surprised myself by feeling sympathetic to the smokers since they have no place else to go. Officials should provide a space for them away from the entranceways. And why on earth was that couple arguing in front of everybody?*

Commentary: Notice that the "good" examples are more detailed and lengthy and avoid making assumptions about people's status or behaviors. As we move to inference and interpretation, specificity and concreteness give way to cautious abstraction and interpretation, gradually inviting in "outside" ideas and information. The personal journal entries are the place to let the reactions and opinions flow—and then reflect on what they mean, to ensure that they do not bias the study.

The average field notebook is not scintillating reading—it will appear long and tedious to an outside reader. At times, the burden to record as much as possible can be onerous; most ethnographers have at least one story of hiding from an informant to avoid yet another encounter. After all, a 15-minute conversation might turn into an hour or more of write-up.

Uses of Video and Photography

Field note taking in real time can divert attention away from observation (Agar, 1980). A question often arises at this point: What about video and photography as ancillary means of observation or as stand-alone methods of data collection? Film and video were pioneered by Margaret Mead and Gregory Bateson during their fieldwork in New Guinea in the 1930s. As presentational forms, ethnographic films such as the 1920s classic *Nanook of the North* and Frederick Wiseman's *Titicut Follies* in 1967 chronicled the decline of traditional culture on the one hand and the horrors of insane asylums on the other. The ubiquity of digital video capacity makes videotaping a readily available companion to field notes for anyone with a cellular phone or video camera. However, use of videotaping and photography presents special legal and ethical issues. Compared to audiotaping, it is much easier to violate a person's privacy because visual images are more identifying and exposing than voice recordings.

The combination of privacy laws and human subjects protections requires that signed releases and informed consent be obtained from all persons in advance of photographing or videotaping them. Some study participants may want to be identified and credited, and this can be an option if anticipated.

Photovoice or *photo elicitation techniques* offer an appealing option that enables study participants to control the camera and tell the story themselves (Carlson, Engebretson, & Chamberlain, 2006; Wang & Redwood-Jones, 2001). Similar to (and often part of) CBPR, photovoice was influenced by the emancipatory writings of Paolo Freire. Its implementation is a means for individuals and communities to document their strengths as well as their concerns in order to effect positive change (Wang, Morrel-Samuels, Hutchinson, Bell, & Pestronk, 2004). Although still needing to adhere to human subjects protections and obtain signed releases, photovoice projects in health promotion and community empowerment have provided valuable opportunities to democratize research practices and achieve collective action (Carlson et al., 2006). Their powerful "every picture tells a story" quality is especially useful in working with communities having low levels of literacy or residents who speak multiple languages and dialects. Gotschi, Delve, and Freyer (2009), for example, used disposable cameras and focus group discussions to understand how social capital emerges from cooperative groups of rural farmers in Mozambique.

In keeping with a participatory ethos, photovoice projects usually incorporate one or more public forums as part of their presentation of findings. As well, annotated photos and videos may be posted on an Internet website for wider access and are key components of the published reports and articles that are produced (and often jointly authored) by members of the project team.

Visual media offer a persuasive tool for informing and advocating, whether the audience is the general public or policy makers or both. In their photovoice study, Wang and colleagues (2004) worked with youths in Flint, Michigan, to document their concerns about neighborhood violence. Their choice of a photo of a school bus window with a bullet hole conveyed a message that words could not capture adequately. As described in Box 6.2, the technique was also used to advocate for addressing health concerns among rural women in Guatemala.

Box 6.2   **Photovoice in Action: Sensitivity to Culture**

Cooper and Yarbrough (2010) employed photovoice and focus groups to better understand health problems from the perspectives of *comadronas,* or birth attendants, living in the rural highlands of Guatemala. Using a sequential "tell me, show me" format, the research team, which consisted of bilingual nurses and research assistants, convened a focus group of 15 women at a local health clinic. The consent forms were verbally reviewed with the women on an individual and group basis (as only 8 of the 15 were able to sign their names on the form). Food and child care were provided for women who had to travel from distant villages. Incentives requested by the participants consisted of work supplies: latex gloves, umbilical clamps, adhesive bandages.

The focus groups were a time-intensive task, as translators worked with the women to ensure all had a chance to speak and be understood correctly. Focus group questions about health concerns of women and children also formed the basis of the "show me" photovoice phase of the project. For this, a subsample of 6 women was nominated by the district nurse as being more capable of using a camera. Two disposable cameras were given to each woman, one for personal use and the other accompanied by a request that she take photos that illustrate her perspectives on health in her community—whether positive or negative. Eleven of the original 15 focus group participants were able to attend a subsequent discussion about the photographs as displayed and explained by the women. The findings from the study noted the women's agreement regarding the health problems shown visually—sanitation (livestock near a water hole), elders' needs (older women tending to their grandchildren), and child labor (young children hauling firewood). Serendipitously, the researchers also observed that young children were given coffee during breaks even though juice or milk was available. This led to a discussion of child nutrition.

In comparing the two modes of data collection—focus group and photo elicitation—the authors conclude that the latter produced data that were "richer, more reflective and more contemplative" due to the advantage of adding visual stimuli to verbal discussions (Cooper & Yarbrough, 2010, p. 650).

Rapid Ethnographic Assessment (REA) and Other Time-Sensitive Methods

Despite increasing demands for time-sensitive methods, the burgeoning literature on qualitative inquiry has been relatively silent on ways to conduct research "on the run." In contrast, the public health literature contains numerous examples of *rapid ethnographic assessment* (REA) and *rapid assessment procedures* (RAP) pioneered by international health organizations allied with anthropologists working in developing countries. Examples include research in nutrition, sanitation, family planning, and HIV/AIDS (Beebe, 2002; Manderson & Aaby, 1992; Scrimshaw, Carballo, Ramos, & Blair, 1991).

REA and RAP are not exclusively qualitative. Key informant interviews regarding the availability of fresh fruits and vegetables, for example, could be combined with a household survey assessing nutritional intake. But REA and RAP are far more likely to include qualitative or mixed methods than to rely on quantitative methods alone.

It is no surprise that the success of time-sensitive methods is enhanced considerably when one or more of the investigators have prior knowledge of the local culture as well as the requisite methodological skills. It would be difficult to imagine, for example, trying to start a family planning program in eastern Kenya (or East Los Angeles) without knowing a great deal about the governmental agencies and health officers involved as well as local religious beliefs, marital practices, and views on women's roles and rights.

The adherence to a naturally evolving, often unpredictable timeline is a defining characteristic of qualitative inquiry. Yet REA and other time-sensitive techniques are often the best and only option for public health research, their salience resting on a sturdy foundation of qualitative methods conducted with as much expertise and time as allowable.

Box 6.3   Rapid Assessment Procedures on the Mexico–U.S. Border

Cifuentes, Alamo, Kendall, Brunkard, and Scrimshaw (2006) carried out a study of sanitation problems and high rates of enteric disease on the U.S.–Mexico border. As part of an initiative promoting clean water in several border towns, local officials sought to understand from residents how and why a community-based environmental intervention was not working as expected. RAP was chosen as the most appropriate and affordable option.

The study began with training of fieldworkers and proceeded with a multi-pronged approach to data collection: informal dialogues with community leaders and local authorities, field note taking and mapping via walkabouts, semi-structured interviews, focus group discussions, and targeted home visits. Fieldworkers were interested in the locations of wells, streams, latrines, and garbage dumps as well as the extent of hand washing, vegetable cleaning, garbage disposal, and water disinfecting. The investigators found that the clean water initiative was threatened by a number of sociocultural and economic factors that transcended individual or household behaviors. Many neighborhoods, for example, were almost depopulated of men who had immigrated across the border to work. Left behind, the women in these communities had less time to give to clean water practices and less income to purchase water disinfectant tablets. Residents offered a number of suggestions for improving the uptake and sustainability of the intervention in the future. The authors conclude that a more participatory approach at the outset would have made the adoption of the clean water program proceed more smoothly.

Summary and Concluding Thoughts

In qualitative studies, the "field" can be a particular site (or sites), the nexus of experiences shared by a group of individuals, or both. Regardless of the form it takes, entering the field requires careful planning amidst near certainty that things will not work out as planned. Earning the trust of study participants and establishing rapport are necessary preconditions to navigating through such uncertainty. Working without the protective layers of distance and presumed neutrality, the qualitative researcher-as-instrument must maintain a level of vigilance toward others as well as toward the self. One enters the field mindful not only of the physical presentation of self (e.g., dress and demeanor), but also of the many identities that may come into play. Personal disclosure by the researcher is a natural consequence of the give-and-take that often occurs before and after an interview (preferably not during).

The immersion and intensity of qualitative inquiry make observation a natural and necessary part of data collection despite its lower visibility in the ever-growing corpus of interview-intensive and interview-only studies. At a minimum, such studies are enhanced by recording observational data surrounding the interview, including the interviewee's nonverbal behavior and the interview setting. Adding a request to "shadow" interviewees can enrich understanding by extending beyond verbal renditions of events.

When the study is focused on a specific place, observation becomes crucial. Whether the researcher acts fully or partially as a participant, the concern is with being as unobtrusive as possible and taking deeply descriptive field notes. Observing can cause understandable trepidation among novice and experienced researchers alike. Practicing the art and science of field note taking is the only way to learn this important skill.

Can an observer fully achieve an insider perspective on what is happening in the field? There is bound to be an impact on what is being observed and what gets recorded, and the researcher must enact a particular role even as rapport and familiarity build. Observation in general and field notes in particular have been criticized as biased and incomplete (Tjora, 2006). Such questions about the nature of ethnographic representation are understandable, but it is the best approximation we have.

EXERCISES

Entering the Field

1. Choose a setting familiar to you such as a shopping mall, day care center, or public park. Think of how you might study it from an ethnographic perspective. Start by drawing a map or floor plan and ponder how this might reflect a

"social order" and affect behavior. Who is the likely gatekeeper? Is there an individual who might become a key informant?

2. In the classroom, do a role-play exercise in which one student acts as a health department administrator and another poses as a researcher seeking permission to conduct a study.

3. Design and print a flyer that you would like to post at a hospital's well-baby clinic seeking new mothers for interviews about child nutrition.

4. Observation in Context

   a. An Hour in the Life . . .
      Spend an hour or more in the "field" as an ethnographer following the guidelines offered in this chapter. This may be in a park, playground, cafe, subway station, or sports arena—any public space where behavior can be unobtrusively observed. After your field notes are written, bring them to class and share with a fellow student. Working together, place brackets around portions that appear more interpretive than descriptive. In other words, try to separate straightforward reporting from assumptions or biases.

   b. Memory Fails . . . Field Note Taking
      Show 10–15 minutes of a movie or video to students and ask them to write a description of what they have seen 24 hours later. Meeting in groups at the next class, students should compare their "field notes" and talk about the selectiveness of memory. Show the movie excerpt again, and then discuss the importance of taking field notes as soon as possible after the observation.

Additional Readings

Agar, M. H. (1980). *The professional stranger: An informal introduction to ethnography.* New York: Academic Press.

DeWalt, K. M., & DeWalt, B. R.(2001). *Participant observation: A guide for fieldworkers.* Walnut Creek, CA: AltaMira Press.

Emerson, R. (2001). *Contemporary field research: Perspectives and formulations.* Long Grove, IL: Waveland Press.

Emerson, R. M., Fretz, R. I., & Shaw, L. L. (1995). *Writing ethnographic fieldnotes.* Chicago: University of Chicago Press.

Gilbert, K. R. (Ed.). (2001). *The emotional nature of qualitative research.* Boca Raton, FL: CRC Press.

Knoblauch, H. (2005). Focused ethnography. *Forum: Qualitative Social Research, 6,* Article 44.

Lee, R. M. (2000). *Unobtrusive measures in social research.* Philadelphia: Open University Press.

Lofland, J., & Lofland, L. (1995). *Analyzing social settings: A guide to qualitative observation and analysis* (3rd ed.). Belmont, CA: Wadsworth.

Madison, D. S. (2005). *Critical ethnography: Method, ethics, and performance* (3rd ed.). Thousand Oaks, CA: Sage.

Manderson, L., & Aaby, P. (1992). An epidemic in the field? Rapid assessment procedures and health research. *Social Science & Medicine, 35,* 839–850.

Prosser, J. (1998). *Image-based research: A sourcebook for qualitative researchers.* London: Falmer Press.

Scrimshaw, S. C., Carballo, M., Ramos, L., & Blair, B. A. (1991). The AIDS rapid anthropological assessment procedures: A tool for health education planning and evaluation. *Health Education Quarterly, 18*(1), 111–123.

Smith, C. D., & Kornblum, W. (Eds.). (1996). *In the field: Readings on the field research experience.* Westport, CT: Praeger.

Spradley, J. (1979). *The ethnographic interview.* New York: Holt, Rinehart & Winston.

Wang, C., & Burris, M. A. (1997). Photovoice: Concept, methodology, and use for participatory needs assessment. *Health Education & Behavior, 24*(3), 369–387.

Wolf, M. (1992). *A thrice-told tale: Feminism, postmodernism, and ethnographic responsibility.* Stanford, CA: Stanford University Press.

7

Interviewing and Use of Documents

T his chapter starts from the realistic premise that high-quality interviews are the linchpin of success for virtually all qualitative studies.
We will carry forward a distinction from the previous chapter by advocating for *interview-intensive* (rather than *interview-only*) studies wherein observation is a source of data even if confined to the interview context. We begin
with informal field interviews, then proceed to in-depth interviewing—
both individual and via focus groups. The chapter ends with the third and
last type of data—documents, archives, and printed materials—then segues
to secondary analysis of qualitative data (a relatively new development in
qualitative research).

Informal Field Interviews

It is fitting to begin this chapter with the type of interview that the previous
chapter introduced—the informal give-and-take that is so much a part of
observation and interaction in the field (Dick, 2006; Spradley, 1979). Such
interviews are context driven and rarely amenable to advance preparation. In
his book on homeless women, Elliot Liebow (1993) explained his approach:

> I was under no pressure to bring ready-made questions into the study situa-
> tion. I did ask questions, of course, but these were not questions I brought

with me from the outside. They are "natural" questions that arose spontaneously and directly out of social situations. . . . They were situation-specific questions, not research questions. (p. 321)

Liebow had many years of experience to anchor such a relaxed approach. Most researchers go into the field with a few starter questions but expect and seek out the impromptu. On-the-spot queries can be straightforward ("Is attendance at group meetings required?") or may entail a brief sit-down ("Can you tell me how patients are educated about diabetes self-care at this clinic?"). Such exchanges with informants allow researchers to gather valuable information and affirm their role as learner. They also serve as the interstitial "glue" that binds long hours of observation with more formal in-depth interviews. Without these ad hoc questions, the informational gaps would make in-depth interviews much longer and more tedious. Informal field interviews may be audio recorded but they usually end up in field notes.

Focus Group Interviews

Focus group methods originated in sociology (Merton, Fiske, & Kendall, 1956) and were developed especially for use in marketing and polling so that small groups of unrelated individuals could be brought together to discuss a new product or political candidate (Krueger, 1994). The size of a focus group should be large enough to generate diversity of opinions but small enough to permit everyone to share in the discussion—about 7 to 10 participants is optimal, but size can range anywhere from 3 to 15 (Morgan, 1997).

As originally conceived, the focus group comprised persons from similar backgrounds who did not know each other very well—because familiarity can lead to more habitual ways of interacting and inhibit fresh opinions from emerging. Focus groups that include persons from different levels of a status hierarchy are considered problematic because the subordinates have understandable concerns about the repercussions of being candid. In practice, both of these prescriptions are violated (Morgan, 1997). In a typical community hospital, for example, it would be nearly impossible to convene focus groups of staff who do not know one another. Less common but also possible are focus groups in which some supervisory staff are included and the topic seems benign enough to allow this to take place.

Focus group interviewing typically involves a moderator (also called a facilitator) who asks open-ended questions, but the degree of direction and structure can vary depending on how narrow or broad the topic of inquiry is. In addition to the need to be sensitive, flexible, and empathic, the moderator must avoid certain pitfalls common to group situations (Fontana & Frey, 1994). These include domination by one person or a clique and lack of participation by some group members. Poor group leaders—those who dominate the discussion or are too passive—can make focus groups a lost cause. Even skilled moderators, however, can find it difficult to channel members away from internal dissension or divisive tactics such as intimidation and ridicule.

The logistics of focus groups require special considerations, both methodological and ethical. These days, scheduling a time and place for several individuals to meet can be a real challenge—early evenings often work best but not always. Inducements such as refreshments usually help with attendance and comfort level. Payment of incentives is also desirable if the budget allows.

The optimal structure of the focus group format is where turn taking is frequent and the moderator exerts control only to ensure a smooth and informative discussion. If at all possible, group moderators should not be tasked with taking notes because their attention needs to be on the group members and what they are saying. For example, MacGregor, Rodger, Cummings, and Leschied (2006) conducted focus groups with foster parents that were cofacilitated by a parent coordinator and university professor, with a graduate research assistant in charge of recording and taking notes. When language differences are involved (as described in Box 6.2 in Chapter 6), a translator may be needed who can work closely with the moderator to ensure that participants are being heard and understood. Although translation detracts from the flow and give-and-take of a group interview, it can be a means of enhancing rapport when done sensitively.

With respect to data collection, audiotaping is commonly used, but some researchers or group participants prefer to have either a scribe or note taker only. Either way, complications may arise when trying to distinguish speakers without revealing their identity—some moderators ask members to adopt a pseudonym or ID number at the outset and use it each time they speak.

As with any method of data collection, focus groups have limitations. An ethical problem can occur when a group member breaches confidentiality. The researcher has no control over this rare but unhappy event, and can only warn prospective group members of this possibility in the consent form. If a group member decides to withdraw from the study, the researcher may be obliged to expunge his or her statements from the transcript.

Focus groups developed and matured outside of the evolving traditions of qualitative methodologies, and their economy and convenience sometimes lead to less-than-rigorous methods (Kidd & Parshall, 2000). Agar and McDonald (1995) raise concerns that "a few hours with a few groups guarantees only that the 'quality' in qualitative will go the way of fast food" (p. 78). No matter how successful, the format of a focus group may discourage going into deeper or more sensitive areas—hence their popular use in marketing (Morgan, 1997).

Despite these potential drawbacks, focus group interviewing can bring clear advantages to a qualitative study, including savings in time and resources and the elicitation of insights from individuals stimulated by the group dynamic. It is particularly well-suited to public health research in organizations or communities where there is a web of social networks already in place. Willis, Green, Daly, Williamson, and Bandyopadhyay (2009) argue that the economic advantages of focus groups in public health research should not overshadow their value in providing evidence to inform practice, whether stand-alone or nested within a larger multi-method study. Focus groups provide a means of group expression and rapport building that no other research technique can match.

In-Depth Interviews

Unlike brief field interviews, intensive interviewing is scheduled in advance, takes place in a private setting conducive to trust and candor, and requires careful preparation. Although there is inevitable variation in how each interview is planned and how it unfolds, there are commonalities as well (Fontana & Frey, 1994; McCracken, 1988; Weiss, 1994). Box 7.1 offers some general tips.

Box 7.1   Tips for Qualitative Interviewing

1. Familiarize yourself with the interview questions as much as possible in advance.

2. Ask follow-up questions based on what you are hearing; use the participants' words when possible.

3. Avoid leading questions.

4. Explore issues but don't interrogate the participant.

5. Feel free to not understand (but don't come across as patronizingly ignorant).

6. Try not to lead with questions about feelings—let feelings emerge naturally and then ask about them.

7. Encourage participants to share anecdotes and specific experiences—avoid generalities.

8. Monitor personal disclosure; emphasize rapport building over drawing attention to yourself (e.g., "I'm a Virgo, too!" is better than "I have the same back pain problems that you have").

9. Don't interrupt or try to control the conversation.

10. Accept pauses as natural; break the silence only if the participant seems stuck.

11. Feel free to laugh and appreciate humor.

12. Avoid becoming informal and "knowing" in follow-up interviews.

13. Take notes for follow-up questions, but don't let them become distracting.

14. Remember that everyone has a "bad interview day"!

In-depth interviews follow different "rhythms of directivity" based on the type of method being employed. Some studies derive their interpretive power from unbroken narratives in which the way a person tells the story is of interest as well as the content of what is being said. Examples include phenomenological, life history, and narrative interviews. In these instances, probes or follow-up questions are minimized to avoid unnecessary interruptions. Other interview methods (e.g., grounded theory) are more dialogic. At the most structured end of this continuum—but still far from the rapid back-and-forth of a quantitative survey—are semi-structured interviews in which the same set of open-ended questions is asked in sequence.

Qualitative interviews are minimally structured, but they are not complete improvisation. Typically, the interview guide reveals the study's key domains (i.e., classes of information from which a variety of questions could be asked, some prepared in advance and others elicited through

probes). Deciding on what constitutes must-have information is important because anything not routinely elicited will emerge only if volunteered or resulting from an ad hoc probe. In the NYSS, we chose not to
directly ask about traumatic experiences because such information was
not essential to the study's goals. We also wanted to respect participants'
privacy and their sometimes precarious emotional state. Although previous research indicated the strong likelihood of traumatic events such as
physical assault and rape, we decided to allow these accounts to emerge
naturally rather than risk appearing voyeuristic. Such information did
come up, mostly from women in the study, in startlingly graphic detail
(Padgett, Hawkins, Abrams, & Davis, 2006).

Interviewing Children and Other Vulnerable Populations

Qualitative interviews with young children are a distinct challenge and
not only because of the ethical concerns discussed in Chapter 5. Young
children lack the verbal abilities, life experiences, and insights that adults
bring to study participation. Older children and adolescents have more
verbal capabilities but may be uncooperative or resistant to questioning.
Highly appropriate for younger age groups is the use of observation (e.g.,
a study of children's social skills in classroom and playground settings).
Irwin and Johnson (2005) offer specific guidelines for researchers whose
studies depend on such interviews.

Persons with mental disability may have advanced dementia, organic
impairment due to brain injury, or a serious mental illness such as schizophrenia. For those on the severe end of the disablement continuum, qualitative interviewing is not feasible. However, the decision to exclude
participants with mental impairment should be made carefully because
stereotypical assumptions can interfere with their right to be heard (not to
mention the researcher's need to learn from them).

Elite and Expert Interviews

Elite or expert interviews may target highly regarded practitioners (e.g., a
famous trauma surgeon), policy makers (e.g., a government official in
charge of health appropriations), or other public figures (e.g., a leading
advocate for persons with AIDS). These individuals add a top-down
insider perspective to a study that would otherwise be missed without

their participation. In what anthropologists fondly refer to as "studying up" (Nader, 1969), interviews with elites require special planning and foresight. Busy professionals and civic leaders have little to gain from talking to a researcher, and some may fear they have plenty to lose despite assurances of confidentiality. Questions usually need to be tailored individually to ensure maximum use of time and to draw on the unique perspective of the interviewee.

The NYSS study design called for interviews with 10 New York City–area leaders in the provision of mental health and substance abuse services. These interviews turned out to be the most difficult to conduct in the entire study. The hassles began with scheduling and repeated postponements or refusals (handled indirectly through a staff subordinate) and continued with the interview itself. With a few exceptions, the NYSS interviewer was questioned about her background and qualifications before the inquiry could begin. Although all expert interviewees eventually spoke freely and informatively, several took time to warm up to the interview process. Once engaged, experts and those in power often enjoy having the opportunity to speak confidentially to a neutral party. More accustomed to journalists who do not subscribe to the same research ethics, they could take comfort in knowing that their identities and associated opinions would be kept confidential. Yet there is one caveat in this regard. It is harder to disguise the identities of experts—the more well-known and opinionated, the more difficult this task can be. Quotes from a well-known judge, an outspoken defender of prisoners' rights, or the director of a large foundation may be revealing for their content alone. Because experts deserve the same protections as other study participants, the use of direct quotes might need to be curtailed in the report.

A Few Guidelines for Starting Out

A qualitative interview is goal-directed. It is conversational without being a conversation, a distinction that is not always easy to recognize or put into practice. A few helpful hints come in handy when contemplating qualitative interviewing. These are drawn from the works of seasoned qualitative researchers such as Weiss (1994), Lofland and Lofland (1995), and Seidman (2006).

First, *clarify your stance* as much as possible, situating it along a continuum of structure and directedness—the phrase "minimally structured" is a good descriptor in most cases. Although study participants are encouraged to see the interviewer as a curious, uninformed learner, the interviewer provides gentle guidance and directs the flow of the interview. It may be a partnership, but the roles remain different and complementary.

Second, *develop an interview guide* well in advance and pilot test it on a few individuals (preferably drawn from the population of interest). As mentioned earlier in this chapter, interview guides consist of open-ended questions structured around the study's domains or categories of informational needs. Keep in mind that vague and ambiguous questions can lead to vague or testy answers (Levy & Hollan, 2000). Thus, a query like "Tell me about your life" might get the reply, "What (or why) do you want to know?"

The spontaneity and flexibility that make qualitative interviews special come from *probes*, some of which can be anticipated and others of which emerge on an ad hoc basis. Interview guides may be standard for all participants, tailored uniquely to each person, or a combination of both standard and person-specific questions. Questions should allow for contingencies such that the interviewer may skip a question that is not relevant or has already been discussed. Giving the interview guide a trial run almost always leads to changes, whether major cutbacks in the number of questions or minor tweaking of wording or sequencing.

Sequencing of questions is very important. Avoid starting out with demographic and other factual questions that give the wrong impression of the purpose of a qualitative interview. Also avoid starting out with highly sensitive questions—save these for later, when rapport is established. The best opening gambit is to ask an open-ended but nonthreatening question, one that engages the study participant without putting him on the spot.

Third, if the study is a team effort, *build in plenty of time for training and supervision of interviewers*, mixing didactic instruction with role-playing exercises. If time permits, transcribe the training interviews and use the transcripts as teaching devices to point out strengths and weaknesses in technique. If time is short, use the early interviews for the same purpose.

Fourth, *plan for the location of the interviews*, attempting when possible to leave this up to the participant. This can present a number of dilemmas because privacy, comfort, and safety are paramount—locales providing all three can be few and far between. Interview sites may include the participant's home, a private office set aside for the purpose, or a quiet public space. In the NYSS, we were fortunate to have centrally located office space for interviewing, although study participants often preferred to stay at home (if they had one). With regard to safety—always a concern but rarely as much as some think—we had an informal policy that no female interviewers would be expected to interview a male in his apartment.

Last but not least, it is always a good idea to *start and end the interview with small talk* when the recorder is not running. This helps produce a smoother beginning, particularly after the dry (but necessary) exercise of going over the informed consent form. At the end of the interview, casual repartee leaves participants with a sense of being appreciated, a chance to pose questions or make comments (including asking for referrals for additional help), and it lays the groundwork for future interviews and contacts.

Conducting the Interview

In-depth interviews have a performative quality in which the players enact their roles while a recorder captures the drama. The interviewer is a low-key presence on the stage, more an enabler than a costar. The "script" is not written in stone; a free-flowing narrative depends on creating space and comfort for the interviewee to speak. Techniques vary, ranging from a quasi-formal back-and-forth to the emotional closeness and mutuality of a feminist or participatory approach (Oakley, 1981; Salmon, 2007).

Probes are critical for getting beyond rehearsed accounts and prefabricated renditions. Box 7.2 gives an example of the importance of probes from a previous study in which I was involved.

Box 7.2	**The Importance of Probes Both Planned and Spontaneous: "Air Theory" and Breast Cancer**

In an earlier study in which I was involved (The Harlem Mammogram Study), we were interested in why some African American women neglected to follow up with diagnostic testing after receiving notice of an abnormal mammogram. In the interviews, we asked about their beliefs regarding what caused breast cancer and its spread throughout the body. Almost in passing, a few women mentioned a firm conviction that "air" is partly or fully responsible. An alert interviewer felt comfortable enough to probe further. Respondents obliged by explaining that opening up the body during surgery exposed dormant cancer cells to the air and precipitated their growth and spread to other

(Continued)

(Continued)

areas of the body. During our regular interviewer debriefings, we agreed that this unforeseen information should be gently probed for because it could shed new light on why women do not follow up on recommendations for surgical biopsies and other diagnostic services. We preferred contextual probes rather than direct questioning; the latter might be perceived as too leading or presumptive. Subsequent interviews and probes revealed varied forms of "air theory" attributions among several of the women, all sharing a general concern with the dangers of ambient air during surgical procedures. A couple of years later, in a surprising twist of fate, this potentially harmful "folk belief" turned out to have more credence than previously thought. In short, it received the biomedical seal of approval when surgical researchers at Columbia University reported that airborne pathogens may explain the greater recurrence of cancer after open-incision surgery compared to closed-incision (laparoscopic) surgery!

Lofland and Lofland (1995) recommend appending facesheets and interviewer reaction sheets to the interview guide. The *facesheet* is a standardized document for recording the date, time, and location of the interview as well as the demographic characteristics (age, sex, race, ethnicity, etc.) of the informant. The *interviewer reaction sheet* is a place to log observations about the interviewee (the informant seemed hostile, distracted, overly eager to please, etc.) and about the setting (the informant's home was immaculately kept; the clinic waiting room was chaotic; etc.). It is also valuable to jot down any concerns about the participant and ideas to follow up. Box 7.3 provides an example of an Interview Feedback Form (IFF) from the NYSS (with some facts changed to shield the participant's identity).

As shown in Box 7.3, interviewer observations capture many things unsaid. Tone of voice (sarcasm, sadness, lightheartedness), speech impediments, facial expressions (grimaces, winks, smiles), body language, and the ambience of the setting (noise, filth, interruptions) provide a feeling for the context that is missing from the transcript if not otherwise noted.

Here are a few additional examples of nonverbal information provided by NYSS interviewers:

- A male participant reenacted a botched robbery attempt in which he had stuck his finger under his jacket to mimic a gun (both in the original incident and during the interview).

- A female participant acted out her newfound pleasure at having her own apartment by gesturing (e.g., unlocking the apartment door, opening her refrigerator).
- A male participant insisted that he was socially isolated even as friends and neighbors stopped by repeatedly during the interview in his apartment.
- A female participant's words were slurred, but it was due to missing teeth and overmedication, not inebriation.
- A male participant kept nodding off during the interview because he had just received his methadone dose.
- A male participant was often sarcastic in tone (e.g., "I'm really popular with women" meaning quite the opposite).

Whether it is the kinetic joy of having one's own apartment or the tone of voice that belies what the speaker is saying, nonverbal communication is an essential part of qualitative research. Box 7.4 offers a psychological rationale for face-to-face interviewing being essential to observing as well as to listening.

What if the respondents' words contradict their actions and circumstances? Take, for example, the respondent described in Box 7.3, who denied having a problem with alcohol despite evidence to the contrary. (In trying to recontact him, we found out from a neighbor that he had died from an alcohol-related illness.) In these instances, it is best not to point out the discrepancy or force a confrontation over what version of events is the "truth." Prolonged engagement with respondents will likely bring this out in time (although a briefer relationship might leave the researcher guessing). In any event, such observations of participant discrepancy need to be noted—a narrow reliance on verbatim transcription would lose this valuable information.

Box 7.3   An Example of Interviewer Feedback From the NYSS

NYSS Interview Feedback Form

(Note: This form should be filled out soon after the interview and brought to the weekly debriefing meeting. If possible, a typed transcript should be included.)
Participant ID #___000_____ M / F_ M_____ Age___47_____
Race/ethnicity ___White (Eastern European)_ Date of Interview_ 03/09/06__
Site of Interview ___NYSS office___ Interviewer_ CA
Time begun_4:00_ Time ended_5:30_

(Continued)

(Continued)

1. **Note study participant (SP)'s demeanor and mood during the interview (anxious, impatient, relaxed, angry, etc.).**
   Emotional, but within reason. SP is an expressive, animated individual. At times he spoke quickly, passionately, and loudly (e.g., about the war in Iraq, other political causes, & his many conspiracy theories). He seemed quite sad when discussing his diabetes and physical pain. He expressed no emotion when discussing other people (family, girlfriend, therapist, etc.). All did not seem important to him. Overall he had an air of fatalism or bleakness—he lacked hope that anything can change (e.g., "I'm going to die here," "No one cares about a crazy old man," etc.). SP was always very warm towards me and at the end, he said "I love you," thanked me profusely for the chance to "tell these things to someone," and asked for another interview.

2. **Note observations of SP's posture or nonverbal behavior. (Remember to include gestures, expressions, and utterances such as laughter or crying in transcript!)**
   Constant gesturing throughout the interview. Mostly hand gestures to emphasize points. In addition, I recall SP showing the size of his room to be about 12′ × 12.′ He showed the pain in his body as beginning in his right foot and going all the way up his right side to his head, and then back down again.

3. **If the interview took place at SP's home: note physical setting, orderliness, personal artifacts such as photos, and so on.**
   Not applicable, but he did have a "Power Puff Girls" (child's) backpack although he does not have children. Also, at one point we were discussing what he likes to do and he pulled an art museum brochure from his backpack. It was addressed to him at the SRO where he is staying.

4. **Summarize briefly SP's history of drug/alcohol use and current status.**
   SP claimed to have no problems with alcohol or drugs. Said he will smoke an occasional joint if he encounters someone with one, but that he doesn't have a problem. Doubt if he is being truthful about ending his long-term alcohol use but did not press him on this.

5. **What (if any) service contacts appeared to be more successful in terms of engagement and retention in care for mental health or substance abuse treatment?**
   None. SP claimed never to have had a problem with substances. He saw a private therapist for a long time but he is not currently attending treatment.

Probes: An Essential Part of the Qualitative Interview

For some interviewees, one question will release the floodgates, but most qualitative interviews rely on probes to obtain the depth and richness desired. As follow-up questions predicated on earlier answers, probes can be used to

- *Go deeper* ("Can you tell me more about . . .?").
- *Go back* ("Earlier you mentioned _____. Please tell me . . .").
- *Clarify* ("And were you homeless when you were arrested?").
- *Steer* ("That's very interesting, but can we return to . . .?").
- *Contrast* ("How would you compare your experiences in foster care with living with your adoptive family?").

Each of these types of probes has a role depending on what is being said and what is being sought. The "go deeper" probe usually opens the door wider than the others. Here, the interviewer must avoid gratuitous questions that can appear voyeuristic if not part of the study's goals and the interview's flow. Probes about sexual functioning can be appropriate if part of a discussion about the side effects of antipsychotic medications but inappropriate if brought up with young adults talking about their dating experiences.

The "steering" probe is used judiciously so as not to interrupt the flow. Respondents are known to go off on tangents, some of which might later yield nuggets of insight while others are yawn inducing. Steering probes come into play when time grows short and content becomes thin.

Less commonly used are *prompts* (i.e., suggested options offered when a question is vague but a "checklist" approach is not appropriate). In the NYSS, we asked participants if they had used health services and then prompted them by mentioning "clinic visits, emergency rooms, and the like" to illustrate what we were after. Obviously, care needs to be taken in using prompts because they may put words in a respondent's mouth.

Should probes be built into the interview guide or emerge spontaneously during the interview? Most studies balance both approaches, planning for some probes in advance but giving the interviewer the latitude to improvise on the spot. A qualitative study that relies on multiple interviewers must ensure that such improvisation does not introduce "solo performances" by interviewers keen on making their stylistic mark.

Developing the Interview Guide

Most qualitative studies implicitly or explicitly rely on domains or topical areas organized around the study's conceptual framework. The following are two examples of domains from the NYSS and sample questions and probes associated with each. In the interview guide, we put the probes in italics to remind the interviewer that they were to be asked only if the interviewee did not cover that information spontaneously. Note that one of the probes also comes with a prompt and that "SP" means "study participant."

Domain: Entering the Program

Sample Question #1: How did you get to this program?

Probe for

- Source of referral
- Degree of choice in entering the program
- If SP was homeless prior to coming to program

Domain: Social Networks

Sample Question #1: Who if anybody can you count on the most to help when you need it?

Probe for

- Relationship to SP
- What type of help do you get from this person?
- Prompt: financial help, child care, food, cash, other
- How they respond when asked for help by SP

Sample Question #2: Is there anyone who counts on you for help?

Probe for

- Relationship to participant
- Type of help given

Sample Question #2 ("Is there anyone who counts on you for help?") almost got left out given the prevailing mind-set regarding persons with serious mental illness as "burdens." It was at first considered a probe under Sample Question #1 but subsequently earned its way to full question status. The usual rule is to upgrade a probe to a question if it is "must have" information that cannot be left to discretion. As it happened, this question not only revealed neglected facets of participants' lives but also helped enhance rapport by signaling that the interviewers were not focused one-sidedly on problems and woes.

When developing an interview guide, pay close attention to the wording of questions to avoid confusion or leading respondents toward certain answers. Consider a scenario in which you are interested in whether and how participants plan for the future. As with any domain, there are many ways to ask about this. The worst from a qualitative point of view would be a question along the lines of "What are your goals for the next 5 years?" Not much better would be "What are your goals for the future?" (although this might well be effective as a probe). The tacit message here is one that many individuals cannot relate to, especially if they are having personal problems and find goal-setting language to be judgmental and too direct. In the NYSS, we settled on easing into the subject by asking "What is the next step for you?" A good follow-up to this would be "Where do you see yourself in the near future?" The "next step" question turned out to be a winner for us, giving participants a chance to reflect on the near or far term as they saw fit and to talk about their hopes as well as concrete plans. In the final NYSS interview, we inserted a probe after the "next step" question, asking "And how about the longer-term future—where do you see yourself?"

How Many Interviews? Issues of Quantity and Quality

There are qualitative studies in which one interview per participant is the only option and even a few where this is preferable. As a general rule, however, it is optimal to conduct at least two interviews per person and allow for more than two when possible (Seidman, 2006). A single interview starts the process and builds rapport and forward momentum for the next interview(s). Multiple interviews provide greater evidentiary adequacy (Morrow & Smith, 1995).

Follow-up interviews fill in missing information, but they are also important as a venue for pursuing leads from earlier interviews. In grounded theory studies, this may occur under the rubric of theoretical sampling where reinterviewing or sampling new participants is an anticipated stage in theory development. Repeated interviewing brings engagement and sets qualitative methods apart from their quantitative one-shot counterparts. When using single interviews, the onus is on the researcher to make the most of these encounters.

Matching Interviewers to Respondents: The Effects of Age, Gender, Race, and Other Characteristics

Given their intrinsic nature as interactive and ongoing social relationships, it is no surprise that "discrepancies and proximities" between interviewers and interviewees deserve serious attention (Manderson et al., 2006, p. 1333). Some researchers advocate matching interviewers with respondents by sex, age, race, and so on. Defenders of matching tend to cite greater acceptability and understandability as advantages because certain topics can be more easily addressed. In the Harlem Mammogram Study (on which I was a coinvestigator), we wanted African American women as interviewers to maximize participants' comfort level when discussing sensitive issues surrounding bodily functions, sexuality, and concerns about racism in health care.

Yet it is not easy to anticipate which interviewer characteristics will help or hinder a study. Robert Weiss (1994) noted the following:

> When I interviewed men who were IV drug users, I was an outsider to the drug culture but an insider to the world of men. When I interviewed a woman who was an IV drug user living in a shelter and also the mother of two children, I was an outsider to the world of women, drug users, and women's shelters, but an insider to the concerns of parents. (p. 137)

Using members of the study population and community as interviewers is laudable (and an essential ingredient of participatory research), but it carries some risks as well. Respondents may fear a loss of privacy by speaking to "one of their own," or they may slant their responses to avoid loss of face with a compatriot. For some studies, the effectiveness of the interview may depend on matching, but for most, being a skilled interviewer is sufficient.

Common Problems and Errors in Qualitative Interviewing

Ideally, the qualitative interviewer has (1) a broad fund of knowledge that makes the inevitable departures from the interview questions productive, and (2) the maturity to be patient, to know when to make these departures, and to know when to remain silent. Even veteran interviewers have had that sinking experience of losing control, what can feel like "taking a puppy for a walk" (Steinmetz, 1991, p. 64).

It helps to anticipate some of the common pitfalls of qualitative interviewing. One occurs when the desire to control or lead compels the interviewer to interrupt the narrative flow. Few things are more disappointing than reading a transcript (or listening to a recording) in which the interviewer dominates the proceedings and cuts off the interviewee. Then there are occasions when the interviewee is uncooperative. It is frustrating to sit across from someone who answers questions in monosyllables, then sits impassively waiting for the next question. The interview stops and starts, frustrations rise, and the interviewer feels at her wit's end. In the NYSS, we were mindful of the fact that the $30 incentive was a serious attraction, but tried to ensure that the relationship transcended its pecuniary beginning.

Respondents who resist cooperating can be exasperating, but the best tactic is to remain calm, be diplomatic, and stop if necessary. No amount of information is worth risking coercion (or a migraine headache). If the resistance appears transitory, another interview can always be scheduled.

Finally, inadequate training and supervision of interviewers in team projects can lead to slippage and unproductive improvisation. Either through carelessness or well-intentioned ad-libbing, poorly supervised interviewers can reproduce all of the pitfalls previously mentioned. Interviewers sometimes get a little too zealous in probing, especially when skeptical about a participant's claim. They could also become too familiar, and the interview becomes conversational and veers off the topic. Once, when perusing transcripts, I came across an interviewer who prefaced a question about drug use with "Sorry, but I have to ask this next question." This seemingly minor act of distancing himself from the study sent a message of not taking the question seriously, thereby practically inviting participants to fudge the truth.

During a successful interview, qualitative researchers strike a balance between the general and the particular, the need to stay focused versus the need to probe more deeply. Simultaneously, the interviewer is expected to listen empathically, monitor body language, anticipate the next question, and mentally or literally take note of red flags (e.g., discrepancies, statements signaling deeper meaning). When everything is clicking, both interviewer and interviewee part company feeling they have had a mutually beneficial encounter. Even a less-than-perfect qualitative interview leaves most interviewees gratified by the experience of being respected and listened to.

Emotional Issues in Interviewing

The sensitive nature of qualitative research almost guarantees that emotionally laden information will surface. Study participants may laugh, cry, or grow angry during an interview. Levy and Hollan (2000) write about exaggerating the fragility of the interviewee as a recurring problem for novice researchers (and as well for those in the practicing professions accustomed to being in a helping mode). Sensitive topics and traumatic stories can and do bring painful emotions to the surface; interviewers should never gratuitously probe or show insensitivity in other ways. Yet to avoid addressing this information simply because it is emotion-laden deprives the study and assumes that participants are incapable of handling themselves and their emotions. Indeed, the vast majority welcome the opportunity to tell their story to an empathic, nonjudgmental listener. It is rare that emotions cause more than momentary interruptions.

Human subjects committees often object that studies of sensitive topics will set off a chain reaction of emotional turmoil that harms research participants. Weiss (1994) argues forcefully that the nature of qualitative interviewing works against this. Even when interviews prompt strong reactions, a skilled interviewer can show concern and then gently steer respondents to a calmer state of mind. In any event, the qualitative interviewer does not try to elicit strong emotions, but only tries to create a safe space for their expression if and when they occur.

What about the effects on the interviewer—the backwash of emotions that follows an intensely personal and painful encounter? In their grounded theory study of qualitative researchers' experiences, Dickson-Swift, James, Kippen, and Liamputtong (2007) found that maintaining rapport, monitoring self-disclosure, and dealing with guilt can take their toll. Satisfaction with a job well done may be tempered by exhaustion and numbness. Similarly, González-López (2010) interviewed Mexican survivors of incest and found herself in an unexpected confrontation with her own assumptions and ethnic identity. For example, some respondents reported beneficial effects of incestuous relationships with cousins, and others professed beliefs that molestation by Catholic priests constituted "incest" as a type of familial betrayal and "sexualized pain" (p. 569). Unlike the relationship between practitioner and client, the qualitative interviewer does not have the protection of clinical distance, settling instead for an "emotional middle distance" (Weiss, 1994, p. 123). One important way to maintain this is through debriefing (more about this in Chapter 9). In the NYSS, the team met weekly to debrief about each interview that occurred in the previous week. Although most interviews take place without incident, the infrequent exception is worth discussing further, whether it is a study participant or interviewer who needs help.

Interviewing in a Non-English Language

It is an understatement to note that the rapid growth in global public health has made research with non–English-speaking populations a far more common occurrence. Unfortunately, the methods that provide the smoothest entrée for doing this have come with few instructions for dealing with diverse languages and cultures.

It is somewhat ironic that the vast literature on qualitative methods since the 1970s has been virtually silent on this issue, leading one to erroneously conclude that qualitative research is an English-only enterprise (Esposito, 2001; Shibusawa & Lukens, 2004; Twinn, 1997). Anthropologists, long accustomed to cross-language research, have traditionally relied on translators when they were unable to master the language themselves. However, ethnographers over the decades have often treated language barriers as a technical hurdle unworthy of lengthy consideration.

This neglect can be seen as a consequence of the explosive growth in qualitative methods in the professions in the United States and other English-speaking countries. Working in education, nursing, and social work, qualitative researchers naturally gravitated toward studies close to home, both linguistically and topically The move toward interview-intensive studies also tipped the balance toward monolingual studies. Methods of qualitative analysis became more dependent on deriving meaning from texts (verbatim transcripts in particular), so venturing beyond the English language risked distortion and complicated research designs and sampling.

Qualitative interviewers who do not speak the language of their study participants must rely on translation or include bilingual interviewers as members of the research team. Although some qualitative methods do not work well with linguistic distance (e.g., phenomenological interviewing), most can be used with intervening translation. Care must be taken, however, to reduce distortions and misunderstandings as much as possible.

Interviewing at a Distance: Telephone and Computer-Mediated Interviews

Notwithstanding the vaunted status of in-person encounters, there are occasions when these are either not feasible or not the point. E-mail and other forms of computer-mediated interviews—not to mention the old-fashioned telephone—have risen in popularity in qualitative research (Beck, 2005; Hamilton & Bowers, 2006; Hessler et al., 2003; Hunt & McHale, 2007; Illingworth, 2001; McCoyd & Kerson, 2006). There are, of course, differences between these two modes of communication. Telephone interviews share with in-person interviews the need to schedule the encounter (not so easy these days), but they have the advantage of the possibility of being audiotaped, thus retaining access to voice and intonation. Although there are always exceptions to prove the rule, telephone interviewing should be seen as a stopgap or fallback measure. Ideally, it is reserved for second (or later follow-up) interviews and when respondents live far away or are not available for other reasons. Cell phone text messaging, the preferred medium of young people, is immediate and interactive but has such severe space limits as to be of little use to qualitative researchers beyond brief check-ins.

Internet interviewing has taken on a life of its own, opening new ways to communicate with isolated, stigmatized populations as well as with technologically savvy respondents who prefer the relative anonymity of the Internet (Beck, 2005; Hessler et al., 2003; Illingworth, 2001; Markham, 2005). With the exception of video conferencing, Internet communications such as e-mail or blogs do not need to be scheduled and are convenient for respondents sitting in the comfort of their home, office, or Internet cafe (D. Miller & Slater, 2000). Assuming that appropriate gatekeepers give permission where necessary (e.g., a website sponsor), Internet communications can be carried out with multiple participants from around the world (or around the corner). By allowing time for reflection, they can yield more thoughtful replies (Hunt & McHale, 2007). Notably, they do not incur transcription costs and may be treated as archival data or documents. Beck (2005), for example, used content analysis of online interviews with an international sample of women who had experienced birth trauma. McCoyd and Kerson (2006) took advantage of an opportunity to compare in-person, telephone, and e-mail formats for intensive interviews with women who had terminated a pregnancy because of fetal anomalies. They found several advantages to e-mail interviewing, including (1) obtaining a credible sample (referrals through physicians being less effective), (2) receiving the data in typed form (saving on the costs of transcription), and (3) affording opportunities for the spontaneous outpouring of thoughts and feelings at any hour of the day or night. The same advantages of face-to-face interviewing outlined in Box 7.4 can put respondents on the spot or cause them to feel less safe. In a sense, e-mail interviews give respondents more control (McCoyd & Kerson, 2006). This can increase rapport as long as the researchers can balance freewheeling communication with the need to obtain necessary information.

Box 7.4   The Importance of Face-to-Face Interviewing

In this era of the electronic commons and highly mobile lifestyles, it is tempting to conduct interviews over the telephone, by e-mail, via Internet chat rooms, and so on. Distance interviewing is appropriate for some studies, but it comes with a significant price: the loss of information that comes from an in-person encounter. Psychologists have noted that the brain's orbitofrontal cortex (the center for empathy) modulates the amygdala (center for impulsivity) during social interactions. Such neurological processing depends on a cascade of socially coded cues including tone of voice, facial expressions, and body posture (Goleman, 2007). There are numerous ways that individuals convey meaning during face-to-face contacts—a raised eyebrow, sarcastic tone, a smile, and a wink all have connotations, and these may be further differentiated by culture. Whereas telephone conversation captures some of the aural cues, online communication offers none (hence the use of emoticons). For the qualitative researcher, authenticity and candor are the sine qua non of in-depth interviewing. A study participant is less likely to shade the truth or hold back when sitting across from the interviewer.

The same advantages that make Internet interviews attractive also have a downside. The low-demand impersonal aspects of e-mail interactions make it much easier to falsify or withhold information. In the absence of in-person interaction and visual cues (see Box 7.4), participants may lose interest or drop out without the researcher being aware of their decision (Hamilton & Bowers, 2006; Hunt & McHale, 2007). Concerned, the researcher may succumb to the temptation to make repeated but unwelcome attempts at contact. Another ethical concern arises from the lack of security attending Internet communication, no matter how diligent the researcher is in encrypting or password-protecting them.

Internet communications can be the best or only way to tap into a network of individuals, assuming that they share a propensity to use online support groups, chat rooms, and the like. Of course, online interviews leave out individuals without ready access to a computer or the wherewithal to use one, a bias that tilts against the economically disadvantaged. As with so many options in qualitative research, the decision should be driven by appropriateness rather than convenience.

Use of Audio Recorders and Other Logistical Considerations

Technological advances in audio recorders and computer software have greatly enhanced data collection and management. The superior technology and lower costs of digital voice recorders have made them accessible for most budgets. The newer recorders come with the software to enable one to download the interview onto a computer and transcribe it directly using controls displayed on the screen (with headphones plugged into the computer). Although longed for by weary transcriptionists and resource-tight qualitative researchers, voice recognition software (allowing one to sidestep listening and typing interviews verbatim) is not up to the task of replacing the human ear. Programmed to recognize one voice at a time, and not always accurately, the software is poorly suited for studies with multiple voices (which is, of course, the norm). Audio recording allows the interviewer to concentrate on what is being said. It also has the advantage of capturing laughter, sighs, and sarcasm—aural aspects of the interview that are vivid and revealing.

Logistical concerns relate to the timing, length, and location of the interview. Given the balance of power in the researcher–respondent relationship, qualitative researchers must maintain flexible schedules, operating at the interviewee's convenience, not their own. Some settings tax the patience of even the most dedicated researcher—crying children, ringing cell phones, and other ambient noise can be annoying and distracting.

Fire trucks and car alarms were the background "music" for many NYSS interviews, but our choice of audio recorders—one or two steps above the least expensive—paid dividends in capturing even soft or slurred voices.

Incorporating Standardized Measures Into Qualitative Interviews

A qualitative researcher not averse to mixed methods might reasonably wonder if a standardized measure could be used for one or more of the study's domains. There is a plethora of measures available for all manner of cognitive, emotional, and behavioral phenomena. The inclusion of such measures and indexes usually implies that they are nested within what is otherwise a predominantly qualitative study (as discussed in Chapter 3).

Miles and Huberman (1994) suggest that checklists or measures be used when the domain

- is conceptually important.
- can be unbundled easily into distinct indicators or components.
- is part of a study that needs comparability across cases.
- has the potential for comparison to other studies measuring it in a similar way.

As shown in Box 7.5, we used some checklists and indexes in the NYSS. Yet the decision to do so is not without consequences. First, standardized measures detract from what is otherwise a more free-flowing experience. When used, they should be reserved for the interview's end or a follow-up interview. Second, their quantitative properties introduce numbers into the analyses, even though sample sizes are rarely large enough to sustain statistics beyond the descriptive level of frequencies, ranges, and averages (more on this subject in Chapter 8).

Box 7.5	Checklists and Standardized Measures in the NYSS

Checklists turned out to be useful in Phase 2 of the NYSS for two domains—service needs and markers of recovery. We used a Services Needs Checklist (SNC) to capture participants' perceived needs in a range of areas (housing, substance

(Continued)

(Continued)

abuse treatment, food stamps, etc.). The Mental Health Recovery Index (MHRI) was more complicated to operationalize. We consulted the expanding but still relatively sparse literature on serious mental illness and recovery and found a few measures in which the emphasis was on programs rather than clients (Onken, Craig, Ridgway, Ralph, & Cook, 2004). We revisited the recovery litera- ture (Ridgway, 2001) and the writings of Patricia Deegan, a leading advocate for mental health consumers who recovered from schizophrenia (www.pat deegan.com). From this, we derived several key indicators of recovery, including

- Having a partner or close friend who you trust
- Having a job or way of making a living
- Using psychiatric medications as needed
- Going to self-help groups as needed
- Belonging to a social group
- Being active in society as a citizen

To these six items we added "Having a safe, affordable place to live," because we were studying homeless adults. What is missing from this checklist is something that virtually all recovery advocates agree is crucial—hope (Ridgway, 2001). Although we may live to regret it, we chose not to ask directly about respondents' sense of hope, reasoning that this would elicit socially desirable or inauthentic responses. Instead, we planned to rely on qualitative observations from interview transcripts and interviewer feedback during case study analyses to detect signs of hope from how participants talk about the future.

With or without the inclusion of measures, qualitative interviewing is defined by its intensity and by a researcher–participant relationship with-out parallels in quantitative interviewing. Box 7.6 addresses the effects of qualitative interviews as "unintentional interventions." As with all research interviews, such effects can be negative (although rarely harm-ful). But the empathy and trust in which qualitative interviews are steeped more often bring therapeutic effects that leave participants grati-fied at being able to speak their minds and use their own words. Under these circumstances, negative outcomes are more likely to come from end-ing the relationship than from its continuation.

Box 7.6	Interviews as Unintentional Interventions

A study of vulnerable or disadvantaged persons casts most interviewers (wittingly or unwittingly) as members of a privileged class. In the NYSS, this relative affluence did not go unnoticed by study participants (SPs). Comments such as "I want to dress in a clean shirt and pants like you" or "You're lucky you have nice teeth" are reminders that interviewers' appearance and behavior are an integral part of the exchange. In-depth interviews afford unique opportunities for participants to self-reflect. Sitting across from an empathic interviewer who asks about life experiences and personal relationships can prompt SPs to think about their lives and what might need changing. Sometimes SPs seek to transform the interview into an intervention (e.g., asking for advice on handling a child's misbehavior or getting into a job training program). While overt helping is generally avoided in qualitative interviewing, the very existence of the interviews and the relationships they entail constitute a form of intervention for good or ill. Higher levels of involvement bring more intense relationships. In the NYSS, for example, we interviewed SPs three times over 12 months and conducted monthly check-in interviews via telephone or in person. These encounters were accompanied by cash incentives, and the meetings were respectful and empathic, leaving time for small talk and inquiries about how things are going. SPs often noted to NYSS staff that their study participation constituted a significant event in their lives. It would be naïve to think otherwise—although no such assumption should be made automatically. Still, it is a good idea to address the possibility of "unintentional intervention" and ensure that the relationship continues and ends on a positive note. SPs should be fully cognizant that an end to the study will surely come and promises of confidentiality will not be broken. Likewise, interviewers often need debriefing themselves to deal with the separation.

Using Documents, Archives, and Existing Data

A variety of documents and materials are of interest to qualitative researchers. These include printed matter such as medical records, case reports, minutes of meetings, brochures, diaries, photographs, letters, and so forth. Archived videos, films, and photographs are also useful. Jacelon and Imperio (2005) describe how researcher-solicited diaries can be a valuable source of data in qualitative research with older adults. Similar to e-mail elicitation, such diaries are useful supplements to in-person interviews, permitting at-will entries any time of the day or night.

Pre-existing documents and data have advantages over interviewing and observation, including their lack of reactivity. In contrast, the presence of an observer or interviewer has to have some impact on the natural course of events no matter how unobtrusive one tries to be. Use of documents is also less time-consuming and emotionally taxing compared to observation and interviewing.

However, documents have some disadvantages, especially when not produced for research purposes. They may be inaccurate, uneven, or incomplete. Some of this is due to hurried record keeping, but it can also be deliberate. For example, minutes of staff meetings may be doctored to cover up embarrassing revelations, or a physician may omit mention of a psychiatric history in a medical file to protect her patient from stigma. Clearly, a study dependent on documents and existing research data is constrained by what is available and its quality.

In addition, access to such data varies. Individuals may freely share personal documents with a researcher (e.g., diaries, photographs, letters). Less available are documents covered by privacy protections, copyright laws, and the like. The advent of federally mandated HIPPA regulations in the United States has made one source of data—medical records— retrievable only with special consent from the patient. As with all forms of data, appropriate permissions must be sought.

Cultural anthropologists have long been interested in "material culture" as a way of understanding social structure, religious practices, and the like. Archeologists and historians are accustomed to relying on archives, artifacts, and other physical traces of human activity. Many behaviors leave behind detectable traces—broken windows in a parked car, crack vials in a schoolyard, cast-off fast food wrappers—that are revealing in themselves. These usually exist as objects of recording (presence or absence, location, frequency, larger context) that stand in contrast to "deeper" documentary data such as court documents, diaries, or family photographs.

Internet-based documents and information may be subject to copyright protection, or their use may constitute an invasion of privacy (e.g., online support groups). The threshold between interviewing via e-mail and "existing data" can get blurry. In their study of researcher-elicited diaries kept by adolescents and sent via e-mail, Hessler and colleagues (2003) avoided elicitation and attempted to be as unobtrusive as possible, so the diary entries were aggregated and treated as archival materials.

Given the overwhelming emphasis on interviewing in qualitative research, documents as a source of data have fallen out of favor in much the same way as observation. They should not be considered an afterthought, however. Although not created for research purposes, their advantages in low reactivity and availability offset many such limitations.

Secondary Analysis in Qualitative Research

The explosive growth in the popularity of qualitative research has understandably led to the stockpiling of large stores of data in electronic files as well as in hard copy format. These may include audiotapes, interview transcripts, field notes, and documents. Secondary analysis, traditionally the province of quantitative research, is increasingly an option in qualitative research (Thorne, 1998). Although analyzing existing data does not provide the warmth and good cheer that follow a successful interview or day in the field, the data's ready availability is a viable trade-off (Williams & Collins, 2002). The next chapter will provide more details on this subject.

Ending Data Collection and Leaving the Field

The decision to end data collection depends on a number of factors, both methodological and practical. With regard to the former, closure usually comes when *saturation* has been achieved (i.e., when additional analyses of the data bring redundancy and reveal no new information; Morse, 1995). Borrowed from grounded theory and now used widely, this somewhat vague prescription is often juxtaposed against practicalities such as deadlines imposed by the study's sponsors or by resource constraints. A general rule of thumb on saturation is this: Studies with relatively homogeneous domains or sampling strategies are likely to reach this endpoint faster than those with broader reach and ambition. Discussion of saturation related to data analysis will follow in Chapter 8.

Two aspects of data collection are peculiar to the timeline of qualitative research: the flexibility of the design and the likelihood of return visits to the field (Iversen, 2009). There are also the usual exigencies (e.g., transcription is delayed, participants become elusive, or the researcher gets distracted by other responsibilities). Some qualitative methods, most notably ethnography and community-based participatory research, need longer periods of time to come to fruition. In this context, the relationship between researchers and participants continues, but it may ebb and flow depending on the stage of the study and the availability of resources to carry it out.

As discussed earlier, stopping qualitative data collection can have an emotional component that does not exist in quantitative studies. Study participants may regret losing the respectful camaraderie, and many a qualitative researcher has felt bereft by study's end (although we should not assume that participants need or want us to stick around).

Ely et al. (1991) recommend keeping the door open in the final interview with an understanding that follow-up contacts may be needed. Modest payback in the form of mailings containing summaries of the findings constitutes a way to demonstrate respect in the study's aftermath. Study participants sometimes ask if they can call to say hello or to check on the progress of the study—this is a reasonable request that should be honored even if they choose not to follow through on it.

Summary and Concluding Thoughts

This chapter complemented the previous chapter in discussing the two additional sources of data in qualitative research: interviews and existing documents and other materials. Interviews may be an informal part of ethnographic fieldwork or a sit-down affair lasting several hours. Although typically done via face-to-face meetings, qualitative interviews may also be conducted via telephone or the Internet. This convenience comes at a significant price, however, in the loss of visual and other sensory cues that give meaning to interpersonal communication.

Among types of interviewees, children as well as persons with severely limited mental capacity are less likely to provide the depth and insight that a qualitative study requires (unless it is heavily reliant upon observational data). Persons in power and experts are harder to engage and often reluctant to speak candidly in an unrehearsed manner. Language differences are surprisingly neglected in the literature on qualitative methods, but they merit serious consideration given the potential for distortions and cultural misunderstanding.

Qualitative interviewing occurs in different ways and contexts, but its signature format is in person, individually or in small groups. Advance preparation involves developing and pilot testing an interview guide; familiarizing one's self with its contents; and practicing the gentle art of probes, both planned and spontaneous. Conducting the interview is an exercise in multitasking (i.e., asking questions, observing nonverbal behavior, and unobtrusively taking notes on follow-up questions). Audiotaping relieves the interviewer of the onerous (and error-ridden) task of verbatim note taking. When at all possible (and most of the time it is), each participant is interviewed more than once to ensure depth and completeness.

The third type of qualitative data—documents and other materials—are the tangible and nonreactive by-products of human activity. Documents originate from a number of places, both personal and organizational. Because they were not produced for research purposes, archival materials raise understandable concerns about their accuracy and completeness. Their strengths—availability and naturalness—are balanced by these potential flaws.

Data collection ideally comes to an end when saturation or redundancy has been achieved, but external factors such as deadlines and diminishing resources can also impinge on this. The emotional sequelae of qualitative data collection reverberate throughout the study, often coming into sharp relief as it draws to an end. Safeguards such as periodic debriefings help deal with intense feelings—both positive and negative. Simply paying attention to the possibility (or inevitability) of such feelings and addressing them with sensitivity can make closure much easier for all concerned.

EXERCISES

Exercise #1: Conducting an Interview

This exercise exposes the student to the intensity and flexibility of a qualitative interview. It also vividly illustrates how time-consuming interviewing and transcribing are.

1. Choose a topic of interest and seek out a knowledgeable respondent for an open-ended interview. Develop an interview guide of four to five questions.

2. Conduct the interview using an audio recorder. Make sure it lasts at least 30 minutes.

3. Transcribe the interview verbatim.

4. Share the transcript with others and look for areas of improvement. For example, did you interrupt the flow? Ask leading questions? Become too conversational?

Exercise #2: Using Available Documents: What Can Be Learned?

Think about your workplace or another familiar work setting as the object of study. Now consider that you have been asked to study this site using only documents, archival materials, and so on—no observation or interviewing is allowed. Address the following:

1. Develop a list of the types of documents available.

2. How would you evaluate the relative quality and quantity of these materials?

3. Do you have any concerns about their accuracy and completeness? If so, what are they?

Additional Readings

Atkinson, R. (1998). *The life story interview.* Thousand Oaks, CA: Sage.

Best, S. J., & Krueger, B. S. (2004). *Internet data collection.* Thousand Oaks, CA: Sage.

Fontana, A., & Frey, J. H. (2005). The interview: From neutral stance to political involvement. In N. K. Denzin & Y. S. Lincoln (Eds.), *The SAGE handbook of qualitative research* (3rd ed., pp. 695–728). Thousand Oaks, CA: Sage.

Gubrium, J. F., & Holstein, J. A. (Eds.). (2002). *Handbook of interview research.* Thousand Oaks, CA: Sage.

Hewson, C., Yule, P., Laurent, D., & Vogel, C. (2003). *Internet research methods: A practical guide for the social and behavioral sciences.* Thousand Oaks, CA: Sage.

Irwin, L. G., & Johnson, J. (2005). Interviewing young children: Explicating our practices and dilemmas. *Qualitative Health Research, 15*(6), 821–831.

Krueger, R. A., & Casey, M. A. (2009). *Focus groups: A practical guide for applied research* (4th ed.). Thousand Oaks, CA: Sage.

Kvale, S., & Brinkman, S. (2009). *InterViews: Learning the craft of qualitative research interviewing.* Thousand Oaks, CA: Sage.

Manderson, L., Bennett, E., & Andajani-Sutjaho, S. (2006). The social dynamics of the interview: Age, class, and gender. *Qualitative Health Research, 16*(10), 1317–1334.

Markham, A. N. (2005). The methods, politics, and ethics of representation in online ethnography. In N. K. Denzin & Y. S. Lincoln (Eds.), *The SAGE handbook of qualitative research* (3rd ed., pp. 793–820). Thousand Oaks, CA: Sage.

McCracken, G. (1988). *The long interview.* Newbury Park, CA: Sage.

Miller, D., & Slater, D. (2000). *The Internet: An ethnographic approach.* New York: Berg.

Mishler, E. G. (1991). *Research interviewing: Context and narrative.* Cambridge, MA: Harvard University Press.

Morgan, D. L. (1997). *Focus groups as qualitative research.* Thousand Oaks, CA: Sage.

Morgan, D. L., & Krueger, R. A. (Eds.). (1998). *The focus group kit.* Thousand Oaks, CA: Sage.

Oakley, A. (1981). Interviewing women: A contradiction in terms. In H. Roberts (Ed.), *Doing feminist research* (pp. 30–61). London: Routledge & Kegan Paul.

Rubin, H. J., & Rubin, I. S. (2005). *Qualitative interviewing: The art of hearing data* (2nd ed.). Thousand Oaks, CA: Sage.

Seidman, I. (2006). *Interviewing as qualitative research.* New York: Teachers College Press.

Spradley, J. P. (1979). *The ethnographic interview.* New York: Holt, Rinehart & Winston.

Stewart, D. W., Shamdasani, P. N., & Rook, D. W. (2007). *Focus groups: Theory and practice* (2nd ed.). Thousand Oaks, CA: Sage.

Thorne, S. (1998). Ethical and representational issues in qualitative secondary analysis. *Qualitative Health Research, 8*(4), 547–555.

Weiss, R. (1994). *Learning from strangers: The art and method of qualitative interview studies.* New York: The Free Press.

Wilson, J. C., & Powell, M. (2001). *A guide to interviewing children: Essential skills for counselors, police, lawyers and social workers.* New York: Routledge.

8

Data Analysis and Interpretation

Qualitative data analyses are steeped in choices and decisions. They may emerge from an explicit epistemological framework, or not. They may hew closely to specific procedures or venture into realms of creative artistry. Yet all must contend with masses of raw data that need to be reduced and transformed through an iterative process of reading, describing, and interpreting. Pre-existing theories and concepts may be invited into the proceedings but are asked to stay only if they fit (Charmaz, 2006). The balance between staying close to the data and thinking abstractly and conceptually is a defining feature of qualitative analysis.

Given their origins in naturalistic settings, qualitative methods have an "arts and crafts" approach to analysis. Their localized adaptability has, however, come with a price—a historic tendency to mystify and obscure methods of data analysis. While ethnography has retained much of this mystique, grounded theory opened the door to greater transparency in methods, particularly in data analysis. Legitimate concerns can be raised that such a trend will lead to predictability and staid formulism. However, creativity and interpretive latitude are still what make qualitative inquiry the "art" as well as the "craft" that it is.

Specific forms of analysis cover a wide range of possibilities, from the particularistic (narrative and discourse analyses) to the holistic (case study and ethnography) to approaches falling somewhere in between (phenomenological analysis and grounded theory). This chapter will begin with the logistics of management and preparation of data, and then provide an overview of the separate analytic approaches. Greatest emphasis will be placed on the form of analysis most common in qualitative methods—coding and thematic development.

Data Management: Dealing With Volume Early On

Proper management is essential given the sheer volume of raw data needing storage and accessibility for retrieval. The tasks begin with fully disguising participants (usually with ID numbers) in all transcripts, audio files, field notes, and other documents. When case study analyses are used, an ID number helps to keep the various data sources linked together for each particular case. Inexperienced qualitative researchers are often surprised by the quantity of raw data generated by studying relatively few people. Manwar, Johnson, and Dunlap (1994) studied 80 crack dealers in New York City and generated more than 25,000 pages of text.

Using Qualitative Data Analysis (QDA) Software Part I: Storing and Managing Data

Not surprisingly, computerized versions of the manual filing system of earlier days have become a staple of qualitative data analysis (QDA). QDA software has acquired a must-have status for many researchers, lending technological cachet to a methodology known for being low-tech.

Initially, computerized word processing programs were used to perform the cut-and-paste tasks of coding and analysis, but the popularity of dedicated QDA software such as ATLAS.ti, NVivo, NUD*IST, HyperRESEARCH, and The Ethnograph has spread rapidly. The Centers for Disease Control and Prevention offers a free downloadable version of QDA software known as "CDC EZText" that performs some of the same functions but with less flexibility regarding the free-form nature of many interviews.

The regularity of QDA software upgrades and the learning curve required to use them make it advisable here to stick with a general overview and suggest additional readings and resources including free trial downloads. (See the end of this chapter.) In general, QDA programs work best on PCs rather than Macintosh operating systems (HyperRESEARCH being among the exceptions). However, some programs such as ATLAS.ti can be used with Apple computers, providing they have software emulation. Most of these types of software have a smooth interface with word processing programs, allowing input of documents as well as selected file downloads for printing hard copies. Documents may be in a variety of formats such as doc, rtf, pdf, text, and html (although in my experience with ATLAS.ti, it is far safer to convert all files to rtf format before entering them). Memos are stored separately but can also be coded as text. Innovative features include the incorporation of graphic, audio, and video files and exporting of files to SPSS or Excel. The central functions of QDA software—to store data and facilitate coding and analysis—make it possible to search for connections or hierarchies among codes, to produce graphical displays of codes, and to easily retrieve information in an organized fashion.

QDA programs offer a variety of learning tools including tutorials, online support, and manuals containing screen shots of the program in use. The manuals offer added value by infusing qualitative data analysis instruction into their how-to format (Lewis, 2004). Testimonials from QDA software users invariably agree on one thing: It is imperative to follow the program's instructions carefully. Each program has its own "logic," which may be unfamiliar to even the most computer-savvy users. The decision about whether to use QDA software usually depends on the scope of the project (including its budget) and the researcher's comfort level with learning the ins and outs of the software. A study with substantial amounts of data and multiple users almost always makes the cost of the software worthwhile. A researcher solidly committed to qualitative methods would also find the investment in software a sound decision. Yet many basic QDA functions such as cutting, pasting, and retrieving text can be done manually or on regular word processing programs without this added expense.

Multiple Users and Cross-Site Databases

The standardization of quantitative studies facilitates tasks such as entering data from different sites, managing and cleaning the data, merging files, and making subsets of data available to multiple users. Recently, the rise of large-scale qualitative (and mixed methods) studies has opened the door to similar multiuse scenarios, albeit with some daunting challenges (Manderson, Kelaher, & Woelz-Stirling, 2001). The Three Cities Study, a massive undertaking involving over 2,000 low-income families in Chicago, Boston, and San Antonio, was funded by no less than 7 federal agencies and 14 private foundations (http://web.jhu.edu/threecitystudy). The study's design, which included three waves of data collection and 4 years of ethnography (1999–2003), required the cooperation of multiple investigators and institutions.

The site-specificity and flexible designs of qualitative research seem a poor fit for large-scale collaboration, but it is possible with proper planning and sufficient resources. At a minimum, advance thought needs to be given to coordination across sites to ensure that data sets can be integrated. QDA software can be invaluable for these long-distance transactions. The timing and scope of the cross-site collaboration are key questions that lead to still more questions: Will all data be sent to a central repository or remain local? If the former, when will the data be sent and in what form? If the latter, how will cross-site quality control be monitored? Will full collaboration be activated from the earliest stage of the study or after the data have been collected? How will the collaborative team divvy up tasks? Whereas data collection is inherently site-specific, data analyses and writing may be integrated across sites or take place at a single "headquarters" site. Finally, how will the allocation of responsibilities be reflected in authorship of reports and publications?

Aside from concurrent data collection, multiple uses may occur sequentially as new investigators seek access to archives of qualitative data. As will be discussed later in this chapter, secondary analyses are becoming increasingly common.

Transcribing Interviews

Transcription of audiotapes receives relatively little attention, perhaps because it is mistakenly assumed to be a mechanical task amidst the many cerebral activities associated with data analysis. However, transcription is a form of data transformation that can either enrich or deprive a study depending on how carefully it is done (MacClean, Meyer, & Estable, 2004). The best approach is to transcribe one's own interviews as much as possible and to train and supervise all other transcribers, including making them aware of the need for full confidentiality. Interviewer self-transcription has several advantages, including the ability to (1) fill in unclear passages, (2) insert explanations or clarifications, and (3) obtain timely feedback on one's interviewing technique.

There is no substitute for hearing one's own voice and reliving the interview. For example, an interviewee might use gestures for emphasis or to replace words altogether (e.g., a wink or a smile to mean "I was only joking," a shrug instead of "I don't know," or eye-rolling to signal impatience). Participants often tell animated stories in which they act out scenes for the interviewer's benefit. "Outside" transcribers are left scratching their heads in such instances.

It is optimal to develop basic rules for transcription and ensure that they are followed consistently. These include transcribing nonverbal utterances such as sighs, sobs, and laughter (setting these off with parentheses is helpful). Pauses by the respondent lasting more than a few seconds are worth noting parenthetically. Sometimes the interviewer needs to add a clarifying phrase so that future readers of the transcript will not be confused or misled. In the NYSS, for example, one study participant (SP) spoke repeatedly of "Susie," which led us to think he had a girlfriend, until the interviewer correctly identified "Susie" as SP's dog in the transcript. Sometimes an interviewee slurs incomprehensibly or talks very softly—this can be noted in brackets as [unclear]. Another use of bracketing is to provide translation of foreign language words or idioms.

The transcriber should studiously avoid editing and cleaning up grammar or off-color language. Respondents have a right to have their stories transcribed without cosmetic (and potentially distorting) revisions. This concern with fidelity is not the same as "triaging" transcription (i.e., selectively transcribing to omit tangential portions of the interview). Given time and labor costs, researchers may instruct transcribers to overlook small talk at the beginning and end of the interview or long-winded repetitions of the same story. In these instances, careful supervision is needed to ensure that useful information is not lost.

Here are a few logistical suggestions for transcription:

1. Leave ample margins (for memos and coding), and number the lines sequentially from start to finish.

2. Use a header on every page, noting the interviewer's initials, date of the interview, and date(s) of the transcription.

3. Put interviewer questions in bold font to make it easier to scrutinize the content of questions as well as their length. (Going on too long is a problem.)

4. Start every answer with the participant's identification number so that any chunks of narrative moved to new files will be identifiable; including the line numbers for the moved narrative makes its provenance even clearer.

5. It is usually okay to skip over the many "uhs" and "umms" (the exception being conversation analyses where such utterances are important).

6. Back up all work early and often, and keep back-up files in different places. Although some variant of this story has become the stuff of urban legend, a doctoral student I knew experienced the ultimate nightmare: While in the midst of moving apartments, she had all of her data—original and back-up—stolen from the trunk of her car.

Using "Outside" Transcribers

Given the intense labor that transcription involves, qualitative researchers frequently pay others to do it. This is expensive, but it also saves a lot of time. (Transcribing a 90-minute interview can take 8 to 10 hours and produce more than 30 pages.) If the option to use an outside transcriber is pursued, it should be done with the knowledge that it forecloses the possibility of a close relationship between the researcher and his or her data. One compromise is for interviewers to transcribe their own interviews in the early phases and sporadically thereafter, but hand most of them over to others for transcription.

With regard to remuneration, it can be made per tape, page, or hour. Local norms on this vary. MacClean and colleagues (2004) recommend paying by the hour (rather than by the tape) to ensure full attention to detail. Whatever payment system is devised should be flexible enough to reward accurate and efficient transcription.

Transcribers should be treated as members of the research team whenever possible (Gregory, Russell, & Phillips, 1997). Often drawn from the ranks of graduate students and the underemployed, transcriptionists play key roles in protecting confidentiality and in making decisions about what gets transcribed and how. Interviews are entertaining and informative, but they can also be intensely personal—listening to teary accounts or hate-filled harangues can take its toll. Although the vast majority of qualitative interviews resolve such emotions by the end, transcribers may feel genuine concern toward a participant. Assurances that the study has procedures for making referrals for counseling and that most interviews are quasi-therapeutic (or at least do no harm) are essential. Like other members of the team, transcribers can benefit from periodic debriefing to express their concerns and offer comments.

Protecting Confidentiality During Transcription

Whether given verbally or via a signed form, transcriptionists must promise to maintain strict confidentiality. This still leaves open the question of how much identifying detail should be retained in the transcript. Using identification numbers for study participants does not eliminate the overall risk of breaching privacy because interviewees often refer to others by name during an interview or talk explicitly about programs and places they have experienced. At the same time, instructing transcribers to disguise all names (e.g., by typing only the first letter) removes valuable information from later analysis. In New York City, for example, Lincoln Hospital in the Bronx is a very different place from Lenox Hill Hospital on Manhattan's East Side. Similarly, an SP may mention a particular provider whose name comes up in other interviews as an unusually caring individual. Transcribing verbatim the names of jails and prisons where SPs served time also conveys important information. Although it is clearly essential to fully disguise all names in public presentations of the data and findings, it is better to retain such details in the transcripts.

Human error is a constant factor in transcription. In addition to encountering unfamiliar terminology, transcriptionists may fill in the blanks when the speech is muffled or background noise intrudes. They may decide to edit out foul language or "mispronunciations." Sometimes it is difficult to know who is responsible for the "errors" in a transcript— the transcriber or the interviewee (see Box 8.1).

Box 8.1   A Brief Quiz on Transcription "Errors"

Interviewees may use colorful phrasing and transcribers may err in capturing them or (worse) deliberately change the language. The following quotes contain some examples of transcriber error interspersed with actual statements made by study participants in the NYSS. Can you detect which is which? (The Answer Key follows.)

1. "I was diagnosed as schizo-defective."

2. "The doctor kept saying 'take a seat,' 'take a seat,' and I didn't want to hear 'take a seat.'"

3. "I want to stay at the Plasma Hotel."

4. "I am very bi-popular."

5. "My boyfriend was built like a brick tree-house."

Answer Key: #1, #3, and #5 were actual statements made by participants; #2 and #4 were transcriber errors. Comment #2 should read "Hep C" (hepatitis C) instead of "take a seat," and #4 should read "bipolar" instead of "bi-popular."

Translating From a Non-English Language

As discussed in the previous chapter, the post-1970s literature on qualitative methods has been relatively silent on the issue of non-English translation (Esposito, 2001). In ethnography, prolonged immersion leaves time to correct misunderstandings or inaccuracies, and the risks of distortion by the translation are lower. In contrast, grounded theory and other language-based methods rely heavily on transcripts of interviews that have been filtered twice—once by translation and again by transcription. In this context, use of qualitative data in a non-English language raises a host of new questions not only about the accuracy of translation, but also about its timing relative to transcription and textual analysis (Shibusawa & Lukens, 2004).

Errors in translation can result from a lack of familiarity with local dialects and meanings as well as deliberate (if well-intentioned) bias. Translators may feel that they need to safeguard their community values (e.g., a Spanish-speaking translator decides to leave out embarrassing details about sexual activities recounted by a Puerto Rican woman). Even conscientious and thorough translation cannot capture the nuanced meanings embedded in language. In addition to culture-bound idiomatic phrases, meaning arises from the texture of speech—the words, cadences, and inflections that non-native speakers often fail to understand. For example, the Japanese term *amae* has no English counterpart in its connotation of interdependency and indulgence on the part of siblings caring for an ailing brother or sister (Shibusawa & Lukens, 2004). Concerns about literal translation are further compounded by the inevitable nonverbal cues sent by facial expressions, body language, and so on. As noted by anthropologist Clifford Geertz (1973), a wink may have many cultural and situational meanings, or it may just be an involuntary twitch.

Identical to earlier recommendations regarding transcribers, translators should be included in the research team as full members. They, too, are privy to the intense human emotions evoked by qualitative interviewing and may benefit from debriefing. In addition, sharing a deeper understanding of what the study is about helps transcribers to reduce errors and makes them feel valued as having a substantive contribution to make.

Analyzing Qualitative Data:
The Search for Meaning

Some qualitative researchers assert that findings are discovered (as if they are lying in wait), and others say that findings are social constructions. Beneath this semantic and epistemological divide is a common substrate of activities that involve pattern recognition and thematic development (Boyatzis, 1998; Patton, 2002; Ryan & Bernard, 2003). Such activities are influenced by whether the study is concerned with change over time and whether its "cases" (individuals or other units of analysis) are treated holistically or as part of an aggregate whose words or utterances constitute the raw material of analysis.

Although all data are filtered in some way, qualitative data can be viewed as existing on a continuum based on the degree of abstraction and processing involved. Raw data include field notes, audiotapes, and visual media such as photographs and documents; partially processed data refer to transcripts, translations, and interviewer observations. For many qualitative studies, the next level of processing involves codes—concepts or meaning units drawn from raw and partially processed data—followed by themes or categories. Parallel to data analysis and transformation are auditing and operational tasks including memo writing of analytic decisions and journal keeping to record the researcher's personal reactions, biases, and concerns.

Boyatzis (1998) distinguishes between manifest and latent analysis, the former referring to surface description and the latter to an interpretation of underlying or hidden meaning(s) that goes beyond description. One does not usually plunge into analyzing the latent before gaining a comprehensive understanding of the manifest. Ethnographers, for example, stay at the descriptive level for a long time in order to make their interpretations "deep" and "thick" enough to uncover the tacit meanings of cultural beliefs and practices.

Whereas some methods offer specific (albeit flexible) guidelines for data analysis, others are less explicit in the how-to aspects. Still other qualitative approaches, such as case studies and ethnography, exist as "meta-methods" (i.e., they are broad enough to incorporate differing modes of data collection and analysis). Regardless of approach, qualitative analyses depend on close and careful readings of texts, multitasking to attend to what and how something is said or done, and using filters and analytic axes to organize the process as it unfolds. Qualitative data analysis rarely follows a predictable course, so keeping track of its progress via memo writing is critical.

Use of Case Summaries and Data Displays

Most researchers are familiar with coding as the gateway to data analysis, but there are additional ways to get a handle on one's data. Miles and Huberman (1994) discuss two basic types of data display techniques—matrices and networks. The former consist of rows and columns, and the latter is a series of nodes with links in between. Although superficially similar to quantitative approaches such as cross-tabulations and path analyses, qualitative data displays use narrative or text rather than numbers. Both are used to facilitate visual inspection in the search for patterns and connections.

Case summaries, another heuristic device, involve assembling and summarizing all available data about each particular case so that they may be viewed holistically. A useful option in any qualitative study, case summaries are essential to early stages of case study analysis. They can take the form of stories or vignettes, but they may also be structured around the study's topical domains. Study participants volunteer a lot of information—some important and some not; the case summary organizes this for greater retrievability. In the NYSS, for example, case summaries could be readily consulted to find out how many children a participant had, current substances being abused (if any), and so forth.

When constructing matrices, there is the risk of losing important information—even a densely packed matrix locks the data into a small number of dimensions. Qualitative studies that focus on group comparisons or discrete events have an analytic axis built into their design, but others might be more fully inductive. Problems arise when researchers try to shoehorn data into matrices that do not fit the format, thereby sacrificing nuance and deeper meanings. As noted by Walker and Myrick (2006), the conditional matrices used by Glaser and Strauss (1967) could also be used later in grounded theory analysis.

Theories and Concepts in Qualitative Data Analysis: A Continuum of Involvement

As discussed in Chapter 1, theories and concepts play an important but often misunderstood role in qualitative research. During data analysis, their role is that of informing without determining, lending concepts and ideas without imposing them. Charmaz (2006) aptly refers to "theorizing" as the optimal description of what goes on during qualitative data analysis.

The most prepackaged stance toward concepts and theories conforms to what Crabtree and Miller (1999) call a *template approach*. Using this approach, a researcher relies on a codebook largely or entirely developed in advance. Content analysis is closely associated with this option, but any qualitative study that needs to follow a prescribed conceptual grounding may go this route. At the other end of the continuum are studies that reject the use of pre-existing concepts in favor of naïve immersion in the data. A phenomenological approach, for example, places high priority on exploring the lived experience *de novo* (over again) to reduce filtering and distortion that can undermine authenticity.

Along the continuum's middle ground lie most qualitative studies, especially those using grounded theory. In these instances, the researcher may use sensitizing concepts from existing theories, but their place in the findings is by no means guaranteed. In this way, the sine qua non of qualitative research—its capacity for surprise and new insights—remains intact.

Data Analysis in Diverse Qualitative Approaches

The following are general descriptions of data analysis used in the qualitative approaches that do not depend on coding as their initial means of interacting with the data. Each has its own historic development that is independent of grounded theory and other methods reliant on coding.

Content Analysis in Qualitative Research

Content analysis has a separate and largely quantitative history of use in the field of communications (Berelson, 1952). It was originally developed to quantify the number of incidents of some phenomenon. Content analyses of newspapers, magazines, television, and (more recently) Internet communications could be used to reveal, for example, the frequency of pharmaceutical advertisements, the number of violent incidents involving children, or the prevalence of ethnic and racial slurs in Internet blogs.

Qualitative researchers sometimes use content analysis when examining documents and other textual materials (Krippendorf, 2004). In what bears a close resemblance to coding, Beck (2005) conducted content analysis of Internet interviews to produce themes related to birth trauma. Although the boundaries between thematic coding and content analysis are not always clear, content analysis typically deals with the manifest rather than the latent. Given a choice, most qualitative researchers would opt for an interpretive method that takes full advantage of the depth of qualitative data.

Ethnography and Data Analysis

Regardless of whether they are conducted in Samoa or Springfield, ethnographic methods produce a wealth of data that can quickly overwhelm the researcher unaccustomed to multitasking with minimal guidance. The following quote (Estroff, 1981) describes this laborious tradition:

> Working with these materials was a messy, exasperating, and complicated procedure. I began by reading all the field notes and raw materials repeatedly until I knew what was in each volume and where it was, creating a sort of mental map and table of contents. Then, as the structure and order of presentation of topics became clearer, I literally surrounded myself with data. I made concentric circles of important pages of field notes, articles, books, and drafts, and I perched in the middle of these to think, sort, and combine. Each of these circles became a chapter, but only after it had become a shambles. Days were spent shuffling and grabbing, realizing a whole section needed rewriting and so beginning again, or rescuing all from numerous disasters with the paws of muddy dogs who assaulted me for attention. (pp. 33–34)

Estroff's time-honored approach—still used by many ethnographers 30 years later—relied on manual sorting, visual examination, and intense contemplation about what was being observed and interpreted. In addition to field notes, ethnographic data include interviews supplemented with documents and records. They may also include quantitative measures and analyses.

As a meta-method, ethnography encompasses diverse forms of data. Learning how to "sweep back and forth" and "swoop in and out" of the data is one of the most challenging aspects of analysis. A number of ethnographic experts have stepped forward over the years to demystify and instruct, including Agar (1980), Lofland and Lofland (1995), and LeCompte and Schensul (2010). In the end, the best way to demystify ethnographic data analysis is through hands-on experience.

Case Study Analysis

Like ethnography, case study analysis is a meta-method embracing multiple forms of data and analytic techniques (including quantitative) and lacking detailed procedures for its performance. Multiple case study analysis follows the same principles of a single case study but, for reasons of replication or expansion, depends on more than one case.

A primary feature of case study analysis is going "deep" before going "out" (to larger issues and theories) or, for some studies, going "across" (to other cases) (Flyvbjerg, 2006). Doing within-case analysis means delving into historical background and/or exploring the case in all of its complexity. If very little is known about the case or it has intrinsic interest, analysis may focus more on description than interpretation.

Because cases may be persons, entities, or events, analysis plans vary depending on the nature of the case and the data to be collected. Patton (2002) notes that the choice of a "case" may shift during sampling (e.g., from an entire school to selected classrooms or from classrooms to selected teachers and students). A case study may include both an entity and an event, for example, a study of an elementary school in downtown Manhattan in the aftermath of the September 11th attacks. It can advance an argument. An example of this type of case study is Bradshaw's (1999) study demonstrating that the closure of a military base did not produce the predicted dire consequences. A case study may also explore the causes and consequences of a major policy change, for example, the New York City Police Department's shift to a "broken windows" policy of quality-of-life arrests in the 1990s (Kelling & Coles, 1996).

The term *case study* refers to the process as well as the outcome (Patton, 2002). A "case" is unpacked and its contents closely examined, but the parts are ultimately viewed as a whole and in relation to one another. A "case study-as-product" is a comprehensive description built up from immersion in multiple sources of data.

Box 8.2 discusses multiple case study analyses in the New York Services Study with an emphasis on varied sources of data and the decision making that cross-case comparison entails. Figure 8.1 offers an example of one source of NYSS case data—a "life trajectory" of a 53-year-old female study participant displaying changes in key life domains over time. Multiple case study analysis presents special challenges to ensure that the integrity of the case is maintained during aggregation. Many of the same methods for thematic analysis and pattern recognition discussed in this chapter apply to multiple case study analyses. As a rule, similar cases are easier to cross-case analyze than dissimilar ones.

Figure 8.1 A Sample Life Trajectory From the NYSS

| NYSS ID: 140 | DURATION ACROSS LIFETIME | | Key2 | continuous → | intermittent ---→ | Current Age: 53 |

FIELDS | **key 1**

Timeline: (1957) 5 (1962) 10 (1967) 15 (1972) 20 (1977) 25 (1982) 30 (1987) 35 (1992) 40 (1997) 45 (2002) 50 (2007) 55 60 65

WORK HISTORY
- educational level
  - commentary: *Attends and Graduates from High School*
- vocational training
  - commentary
- agency linked
  - commentary
- independent employ
  - commentary: *Works at a bank after graduation for 2 years, until held at gunpoint in robbery.* — *Works as a home attendant*

INCARCERATION
- jail
  - commentary
- prison
  - commentary

RESIDENTIAL
- street/subway
  - commentary: *Brief period of homelessness when SP loses her room at YWCA, shifts from friend's houses, and even sleeps in father's car overnight* — *lives on streets, subways, buses 1 year*
- shelter/drop-in
  - commentary: *Park Slope Women's Shelter 3 years*
- structured residence
  - commentary: *Adult Residence*
- supported housing
  - commentary
- own apartment/other
  - commentary: *Lived with parents up to graduation* — *Moves to PA Returns to NYC, takes care of ailing uncle and then moves back in w/father* — *lives with friends in Jamaica, Queens*

NYSS ID: 140   **DURATION ACROSS LIFETIME** | **Key2** | continuous → | intermittent ⇢ | Current Age: 53

FIELDS	key 1	(1957) 5	(1962) 10	(1967) 15	(1972) 20	(1977) 25	(1982) 30	(1987) 35	(1992) 40	(1997) 45	(2002) 50	(2007) 55	60	65
MENTAL HEALTH Tx														
Inpatient admission														
commentary														
outpatient treatment														
commentary								*First diagnosed as bi-polar at women's shelter and prescribed psychotropic meds.*						
other														
SUBSTANCE USE														
alcohol														
commentary				*Begins drinking and smoking marijuana at age 12 to age 54 with one year of sobriety in early 20s. Stopped for 11 months currently*										
marijuana														
commentary				*Begins drinking and smoking marijuana at age 12 to age 54 with one year of sobriety in early 20s. Stopped for 11 months currently*										
cocaine/crack														
commentary										*Begins smoking crack in early 40s. Stops using, but continues to drink and smoke pot*				
heroin/opiates														
commentary														
other				*experiments with LSD and psychedelic drugs in late 60s–early 70s*										

(Continued)

169

Figure 8.1 (Continued)

NYSS ID: 140	DURATION ACROSS LIFETIME

Key2	continuous	intermittent	Current Age: 53

FIELDS	key 1	(1957) 5	(1962) 10	(1967) 15	(1972) 20	(1977) 25	(1982) 30	(1987) 35	(1992) 40	(1997) 45	(2002) 50	(2007) 55	60	65
SUBSTANCE Tx														
detox *commentary*														
short-term recovery *commentary*														
long-term recovery *commentary*														
day program *commentary*														
Peer Support Groups														

Box 8.2	**Multiple Case Study Analyses in the NYSS**

In Phase 1 of the NYSS, we conducted case study analyses of individual life histories to ensure that the sequencing and timing of events were given center stage. To carry these out, we assembled and reviewed the data for each study participant (SP) as listed below:

- Interview transcripts (two per SP)
- Interviewer feedback forms documenting observations of the SP interviews
- Brief case summaries
- Life trajectory graph (depicting key events; see Figure 8.1 for an example)

Writing the case summaries required an immediate decision: Would they track the person's life over time or by topical area—for example, substance use, mental illness, homelessness, and so on? We opted for topical areas, but also focused on chronologies (by topic) with a "life trajectory" chart in an Excel spreadsheet format. These life trajectories showed onsets (and endpoints) of substance abuse, homelessness, incarceration, psychiatric treatment, and the like. This color-coded visual display (we had to decide which colors should be assigned to marijuana, cocaine, alcohol, etc.) compressed a tremendous amount of information into several parallel trajectories. Case study analyses were conducted in group meetings that drew on these trajectories and the other case-specific data. With the participant's primary interviewer acting as the discussion leader and another team member acting as scribe, we sat down as a group and discussed each person with a list of questions as a guide. These questions asked about (1) the sequencing of mental illness, homelessness, and substance abuse in the participant's life course; (2) what appears to have "worked" and "not worked" in terms of services for these problems; (3) traumatic events in childhood or adulthood that appeared to be turning points in the participant's life; and (4) other positive or negative events that stand out in the participant's recollections. Answers to these questions formed a focused narrative for each SP that was then compared to the other case narratives to explore commonalities in the life histories. Echoing Patton's (2002) distinction between a pattern and a theme, we found descriptive patterns (e.g., female child sexual abuse, early teen onset of substance abuse, and an absence of work history and job skills) that were not present in all cases but were prevalent enough to be noteworthy. Themes included cumulative adversity and loss, aging and self-reflection as precursors to cessation of substance abuse, and the "situatedness" of mental illness as one of many setbacks in a lifetime of deprivation.

Data Analysis in Narrative Approaches

As discussed in Chapter 2, narrative approaches bring to the surface the tacit meanings embedded in the structure of naturally occurring speech and talk. Whether following the arc of a personal narrative or the back-and-forth of a conversation, the analyst's job is to extract and interpret meaning (Hyden & Overlien, 2004; Sands, 2004). Data analyses in narrative approaches draw on literary traditions while reflecting a social science preoccupation with social and cultural influences. Narrative approaches fall roughly into two types: (1) analyses of stories that naturally occur during interviews, and (2) analyses of conversational exchanges between two or more individuals in which the study participants may be unrelated (e.g., focus groups) or members of a family or group of friends. The first of these, narrative analysis, analyzes storytelling, plots, and chronologies of events (Riessman, 1993). The second, which encompasses discourse and conversation analysis, examines dialogic aspects of human communication.

Following Labov and Waletzky (1967), narrative analysis involves identifying six elements of a fully formed narrative: *abstract* (summary or précis of the event), *orientation* (time, place, participants, context), *complicating action* (what actually transpired), *evaluation* (meaning and significance of the event), *resolution* (conclusion of the event), and *coda* (giving closure by returning the listener to the present time). A few caveats are pertinent here. First, not all narratives contain all six elements, and analysts may reasonably disagree about what constitutes a coda, evaluation, and so forth. Second, narrative stories may be embedded within a long interview, or they can emerge over a series of interviews (Riessman & Quinney, 2005). Finally, some researchers use a modified narrative approach that is less formal, analyzing participants' narratives for thematic commonalities. Davis, Rhodes, and Martin (2004), for example, describe the "risk narratives" of injection drug users as they attempt to avoid contracting hepatitis C (hep C). Participants' mini-stories of injecting the first time, injecting with (and learning from) a more experienced user, and hearing about a hep C diagnosis are revealing in ways that require they be kept intact.

Analyzing naturally occurring speech can uncover social and cultural influences that structure human interaction. *Conversation analysis* does this by examining turn taking; silences and nonverbal utterances that signal gender, age, and race; and other role-playing that is enacted when individuals speak with one another (ten Have, 1999). *Discourse analysis* is more broadly defined to include texts as well as conversation. Analytic procedures center on spotlighting how larger social influences (especially unequal power and dominance) shape modern discourse(s) (Gee, 2005). Sarangi and Candlin (2003), for example, demonstrate how discourse analytic frameworks can be used to explore discussions of risk associated with HIV/AIDS, cancer, and genetic testing.

Phenomenological Analyses

Phenomenological studies fill an important niche by exploring the depths of human experience, whether this experience refers to living with chronic illness or winning the state lottery. Developed largely in the field of psychology (Colaizzi, 1978, Giorgi, 1985), phenomenological data analyses share a few basic activities. These include synopses of each study participant's experiences ("textural description"), examination of the context and setting of these experiences ("structural description"), and a condensation or summary of major themes with associated excerpts from the interviews (Moustakas, 1994). Before and during the analyses, the researcher explores his or her personal experience with (or opinions about) the phenomenon and seeks to "bracket" or sideline it. A step-by-step example of this is provided by Groenewald (2004) in his phenomenological study of educational programs in South Africa. Similarly, Sanders (2003) offers a detailed description of her application of Colaizzi's phenomenological method to a study of spirituality among nurses.

Community-Based Participatory Research: Analyzing Data Collaboratively

Since the data in CBPR may be quantitative as well as qualitative, analytic decisions regarding mixed methods depend upon the study's goals and design (see Chapter 3). In CBPR, the analytic process involves both researchers and community members, the former contributing technical expertise and the latter both assisting in and steering the process (Horowitz, Robinson, & Seifer, 2009). The actual tasks of data analysis are not assumed to be different in CBPR as opposed to other approaches, but they are inherently collaborative.

Coding and Thematic Development

Coding and thematic development are the most commonly used analytic procedures in qualitative research. That said, there is tremendous variety in how these are carried out and described in the final report. The majority of qualitative researchers stay with description and interpretation without producing a fully developed grounded theory or formal schema encompassing all findings. Flick (2004) asserts that requiring theory development constitutes an excessive and unrealistic burden for many studies, especially graduate theses and dissertations. This, of course, does not preclude theoretical thinking (Charmaz, 2006). Notwithstanding the importance of careful coding and indexing of data, much of what makes a qualitative study succeed occurs over and above these activities, i.e., when ideas and interpretations are put into play (Coffey & Atkinson, 1996).

Varied Approaches to Coding

Coding initially involves transferring chunks of text into conceptual "bins," i.e., it breaks the "data apart in analytically relevant ways in order to lead toward further questions about the data" (Coffey & Atkinson, 1996, p. 31). As noted by Tesch (1990), each chunk or quotation has two contexts, one its origin in the narrative and the other a "pool of meaning" located in higher levels of abstraction. Coding both sets the stage for interpretation and is interpretation (albeit in a very rudimentary way).

At the outset, coding involves close and repeated readings of the transcript (or other text) in search of "meaning units" that are descriptively labeled so that they may serve as building blocks for broader conceptualization. Somewhat like a funnel, coding starts at a descriptive level and moves upward to greater selectivity and synthesis (Charmaz, 2006).

Questions and decisions arise early on (e.g., where code labels come from, to what extent can these labels draw on a priori concepts and theories, the level of detail attending the analysis [think of a fine- versus a coarse-toothed comb]). The answers to these questions depend on the study's overall conceptual framework and design, but some basic guidelines are discussed in the following sections.

Starting Out: Identifying and Labeling Codes

Most qualitative researchers begin with open coding (Charmaz, 2006; Ryan & Bernard, 2000). For the novice, this can seem like working the trapeze without a net, but one need not approach coding as a blank slate (pardon the mixed metaphors here). Grounded theorists refer to *sensitizing concepts* (Glaser, 1978) as providing initial guidance on where to start looking. Thus, a study of persons with schizophrenia would likely consider looking for "stigma," and one examining obesity might look at "body image." Regardless of whether sensitizing concepts are invoked, the researcher approaches the text with as few preconceptions as possible and holds the ones she has lightly.

A qualified exception to this comes from evaluation research and rapid assessment projects where codes may be imported directly from the interview questions, with varying degrees of openness to new information and new codes (Patton, 2002). Similar to what Crabtree and Miller (1999) refer to as a "template" approach, we used this selective format in an evaluation of foster care in New York City (Freundlich, Avery, & Padgett, 2007). Consultation with key stakeholder groups (youths, social workers, attorneys, judges) and the literature produced seven domains that structured the open-ended questions as well as the analyses. These domains were youth involvement, transitioning, recommendations for improved services, quality of placements, safety in the placements, services in the placements, and permanency planning. Such pre-packaged codes permitted us to expedite the study's data collection and analysis yet stay true to the stakeholder opinions that shaped their content. The trade-off—losing the freshness and creativity of inductive thinking—was worth it because sponsors and study participants asked for a quick turnaround (less than 18 months) for the results and policy recommendations.

When coding, one can use the right-hand margins of the transcript to bracket relevant segments and assign code labels to them. Although this may be carried out directly on the computer screen using QDA software, I prefer marking hard copies first (always using pencils with erasers). A few important considerations arise at this point. First, every line of the transcript is not necessarily coded (or code-worthy). Second, a single passage of text may be so rich that it yields several code-worthy chunks of information. Coding can get messy in such instances—sometimes one must literally circle the relevant text with an arrow leading to the code label in the margin. (Right-hand margins can look like traffic gridlock when an interview yields a lot of important material.) Third, codes need to have clear definitions to guide their usage (i.e., what belongs in and what does not). Finally, codes are provisional and subject to change, either through clarification and revision or outright elimination.

Early in data analysis—usually after three or four transcripts—a start list of codes is compiled and applied to additional transcripts. A commonly used approach is to have two persons independently code the first few transcripts, and then meet to discuss their findings and arrive at a provisional list of codes. In this way, new codes may be added and excess codes discarded.

Codes get dropped for two primary reasons: (1) They have too few excerpts (or their content is too thin), or (2) they become merged with or absorbed by another code. A code's staying power is not a matter of quantity. Counting the number of times something is mentioned (or the number of lines of text these items occupy) is largely the domain of content analysis.

After coding a few more transcripts (this number varies depending on the density and richness of the data), the list of codes starts to gel and no new codes emerge. The size of the final list can vary considerably, but it tends to become unwieldy when codes number more than 30 or 40. Less (or fewer) codes can be more.

Code labels should be brief but descriptive. Charmaz (2006) suggests using gerunds (-ing words) whenever possible to evoke dynamic processes. In the NYSS, for example, we used the code "living independently" to refer to occasions when study participants talked about the benefits of having an apartment of their own. (See more about this code in Box 8.6 on pages 188 and 189.)

Code labels may be *in vivo*, emerging directly from participants' words. Interviews with case managers in the NYSS led us to use the in vivo code "working the system" to connote the various actions they use to help their clients. We could not hope to improve on this as a label. Sometimes an in vivo code is the product of jargon that has seeped into common parlance. Thus, studies of addiction might encounter the lingo of 12-step groups (e.g., "people, places, and things" or "hitting bottom").

Charmaz (2006) urges the use of compelling or interesting code labels that will grab the reader. Statements like "I take my nephews to school every day" and "I get medicines for my elderly neighbor when she gets sick" might be coded rather dryly as "altruistic actions" or more evocatively as "helping others." Codes with what Charmaz refers to as "grab" are usually in vivo or inductively derived because their graphic nature cannot (and probably should not) be anticipated in advance.

Documenting and Verifying Coding Procedures: Independent Co-Coding

Optimally, coding is done in the early stages by two (or more) co-coders. When the study is conducted by a team, this ideal can be attained rather easily. But even the lone researcher is urged to seek out peers with whom he can co-code (and return the favor at the same time or a later point).

The challenges arise when dealing with the inevitable discrepancies that occur, especially during the early rounds of co-coding. This is almost always a somewhat messy back-and-forth process of forging agreement amidst well-intentioned and reasoned differences. The balancing act involves staying close to the participants' meanings yet capturing them at a level of abstraction that transcends the idiosyncratic. Co-coding will take a few rounds before a codebook coalesces. Once the codebook is complete, coding goes much more smoothly but must remain flexible enough to accommodate new and important information.

Some positivist-oriented researchers calculate intercoder agreement using percentages or statistics such as Cohen's kappa, the latter designed to control for agreement by chance (Mayring, 2004). This has an inherent appeal, as critics often point to subjective bias and unsystematic analyses as the Achilles' heel of qualitative methods.

Yet the thought processes that go into coding and thematic development are more complex than what can be captured by reliability coefficients. Studies in cognitive science have shown there are limits to the amount of information humans can process, and the complex decision making in qualitative data analysis represents such a challenge (Hrushka et al., 2004). Areas of disagreement during co-coding include (1) what segments are deemed code-worthy; (2) the size of a particular segment selected for coding; (3) the choice of words or phrasing for a code label; and (4) the definition of the code, including what is and is not encompassed by it. It is hard to imagine two individuals, no matter how well trained and like-minded, having concordance along most or all of these parameters. Box 8.3 offers some examples of how qualitative researchers have addressed the metrical demands of intercoder reliability assessment and the complications that ensue.

Box 8.3	**Challenges Attending Intercoder Reliability Assessments (IRAs): Examples From a Study of Japanese American Identity and a Series of HIV Studies**

As noted by Kurasaki (2000), it is much easier to assess reliability with discrete portions of text (e.g., short answers to a standard set of open-ended questions) than with the free-flowing text common to most in-depth interviews. In her study

(Continued)

(Continued)

of Japanese American identity, Kurasaki worked with colleagues to develop a set of codes that were then applied to selected text segments to ascertain rates of agreement for each code. Random selection of transcripts and of pages within transcripts produced 20 pages for each of the coders to analyze using the codebook. Agreement was studied by randomly selecting 10 lines on each coded page and assigning a 1 if the coders used the same code for that line (with a range of 5 lines before and after it allowed) and a 0 if they did not agree. The boundary range reflected the varying tendency in bounding the data when coding, with some coders being inclusive and others more stringent. The percent agreement rate (number of agreements divided by number of comparisons) varied across the 17 codes, ranging from .68 to a perfect 1.00 with an average of .90.

Hrushka and colleagues (2004) at the Centers for Disease Control and Prevention used similar procedures to conduct intercoder reliability assessments (IRAs) in three HIV studies. Like Kurasaki, they opted for dichotomous ratings (0, 1) for presence vs. absence of agreement for each code. For each of the three studies, they analyzed the proportion of codes that exceeded .90 in their respective kappa statistic. Summarizing the experience, Hrushka et al. noted that (1) agreement was low in the first coding round despite having a codebook and training in its use. In one of the reviewed studies (the Los Angeles Bathhouse Study), only 39 percent of codes met the cutoff of .90; (2) multiple rounds of coding were needed to increase rates of agreement. The LA Bathhouse Study required 9 rounds to achieve a standard of 90 percent of codes exceeding kappas of .90; (3) larger numbers of codes reduced agreement and increased coder uncertainty; and (4) interviewer variability had an impact; i.e., interviewers who elicited succinct responses made agreement easier.

Commentary: Both of the above-referenced articles were manifestly quantitative in appearance and in content. When done correctly, IRA inexorably leads a qualitative researcher down a path of variable creation and statistical analyses. Though often telescoped into a single sentence in the report, e.g., "We assessed intercoder reliability and found it to be high with a Cohen's kappa of .85," this brief statement belies the amount of effort required to produce it—assuming it was done in such a thorough manner as described here. Some qualitative researchers find this expenditure of time and analytic effort worth it, but a few questions remain: At what cost are these coefficients of agreement achieved? If many rounds of coding are needed, is this more a process of wearing down resistance than of doing justice to the data? Is the pursuit of 90% agreement antithetical to the negotiated mutuality of consensus coding? IRAs obscure a messy reality and may unwittingly give an impression of precision that is "real" rather than imposed by the methods. For qualitative researchers who value immersion in texts and meaning-making, this veneer of certitude is not worth the effort and, in many ways, is not a worthwhile goal.

As described in Box 8.3, intercoder reliability estimations work best with a standardized set of concrete and delimited questions and answers. Yet most qualitative approaches derive their strength from the opposite, that is, from densely described life experiences not easily segmented for reliability assessment. For these studies, coding is more likely to be a process of consensual validation (Sandelowski & Barroso, 2002). Thinking about codes, discussing and defending them, and reaching consensus are valuable aspects of the process, not something to avoid or tamp down. At the same time, it is important to conduct independent co-coding in the early rounds until the codebook is finalized and there is confidence that solo coders will be able to work without committing significant errors.

Comparing and Contrasting: Memo Writing

Memo writing is an ongoing process in which one documents thoughts and ideas that emerge through interacting with the data. Strauss and Corbin (1990) distinguish among three types of memos: code notes, theory notes, and operational notes. *Code memos* are the basis for definitional statements and documentation of their reason for being. *Theory notes* are a record of ideas and hunches about what is going on in the data. *Operational notes* are placeholders for logistical and other concerns. (Box 8.5 on pages 186 and 187 offers some examples of operational notes.)

Memos are safety zones for discovery and creativity, a place for hunches and conjecture. They may be shared with one's advisor or collaborators but otherwise remain private repositories of ideas. It is important to distinguish memos from codes. Codes are indexical (i.e., words or phrases that "speak for" chunks of raw data). Memos are running commentaries rooted in the data but not intended to directly represent it.

As coding proceeds, the analyst remains cognizant of similar incidents in other interviews as well as the larger context, searching for patterns but also remaining alert to negative instances and irregularities. What grounded theorists refer to as *constant comparative analysis* describes a systematic search for similarities and differences across interviews, incidents, and contexts (Strauss & Corbin, 1994). A constant comparative analysis stays close to the data, but its ultimate value comes from an ability to think abstractly and make sense of myriad comparisons, winnowing through them to note what is meaningful. In practice, comparative analysis is cyclical, beginning as inductive, then becoming deductive, and then returning to the inductive. This cycle can be repeated many times over.

Producing Categories and Themes: Differing Analytic Possibilities

It is customary to cut and paste each coded segment into a separate file linked to its respective code label. (QDA software does this and makes the resulting coded segments easily aggregated and retrieved.) Opinions differ on how much of the surrounding context should be grabbed as part of the segment; the rule of thumb is to take as much as is needed to understand the segment later on when it is viewed out of its original context but not to burden it with extraneous material.

A manual version of these tasks dating back to earlier days involved literally cutting an excerpt from an extra copy of the text and pasting it onto an index card with additional information like ID number, line numbers, and so on. A kind of pile sort technique was sometimes used in which the quotes/cards were spread out on a table and gradually organized by themes. "Splitters and lumpers" take different tacks to categorizing, but the former have the edge because fine-grained categories can always be aggregated later on (Ryan & Bernard, 2003). Although rarely done, thematic development may employ quantification as part of the process. Box 8.4 offers one such example.

Box 8.4	An Example of Quantified Thematic Development

Barkin, Ryan, and Gelberg (1999) describe a deductive–inductive approach to analyzing interview data from pediatricians, community leaders, and parents in South Central Los Angeles inquiring about what doctors can do to prevent youth violence. Given the narrow scope and limited time for the study, the researchers started out with three a priori themes: potential (for doctors to address youth violence), barriers (to addressing youth violence), and resources (for addressing youth violence). These themes were used by two team members to identify statements associated with each (numbering 84, 74, and 41, respectively) made by the 26 study participants. For subtheme identification, this deductive approach shifted to inductive as four coders separately pile-sorted the three sets of thematic statements to come up with subthemes. Three of the four coders were naïve (blinded) to the study's goals. Each statement was scaled 0 to 4 depending on the number of coders who placed it in a subtheme pile. The researchers then turned to multidimensional scaling and cluster analysis to identify the final set of subthemes. The distributions of these subthemes were displayed by interview group to show how frequently pediatricians, community leaders, and parents endorsed them. Although the authors did not use the term, the early phases of data analysis resembled content analysis insofar as they were identifying previously selected phenomena and counting their frequency.

As texts are fractured into meaning units, the resulting code files replace transcripts as the focus of analysis. In what Tesch (1990) refers to as decontextualizing and recontextualizing, analyses of code excerpts involve pattern recognition, drawing on comparisons and contrasts. While doing this, the researcher refers back to the study's research questions as well as the literature—keeping in mind what is known and not known.

There is no consensus on what terminology to use when talking about these interim phases of analysis (Walker & Myrick, 2006). Charmaz (2006) refers to *focused coding* as the time when open codes are winnowed down. Focused codes may result from aggregating a few open codes under a single label. Alternatively, an open code with high salience may become a higher-order focused code or even a theme. Driving this process is constant referencing back to the data and making adjustments to accommodate variation in participants' experiences and beliefs. As an example, Charmaz traces the origins of the code "identifying moment" as a descriptor for pivotal incidents when persons with chronic physical illness are reminded by others of their disability. Originally defined as referring only to negative experiences, the code was broadened to include positive ones as well. Ultimately, "identifying moment" became a *category*, the grounded theory term for a theme or pattern that arcs across large swaths of the data. Herein lies an important lesson: Although most codes serve out their duty in the descriptive trenches of analysis, an occasional one will make the jump to higher levels.

In grounded theory, a third type of coding—*axial coding*—specifies the properties of the category and its subcategories (Strauss & Corbin, 1990). Just as open coding parses data into digestible bits, focused and axial coding starts the process of reintegration by creating a preliminary conceptual framework. In practice, few qualitative studies use axial coding, in part because it is demanding and, according to some, overly prescriptive (Kelle & Erzberger, 2004). The same applies to *selective coding,* a process of selecting and refining "core categories" alone and in relationship to one another (Strauss & Corbin, 1990).

Grounded theorists may turn to *theoretical sampling* to tighten and extend their analyses. Unlike initial sampling, theoretical sampling involves the careful selection of additional cases or settings that will help test out emergent hypotheses. Often guided by memos, the logic of theoretical sampling dictates locating cases for a specific purpose—the refinement of the theory. Consider a hypothetical study of adolescents who drop out of high school wherein a pattern emerges from the interview data (e.g., that boys say their reason for leaving was bullying and intimidation and girls say their family responsibilities interfered with school). Further analyses lead to developing a provisional theory of gender differences in "push versus pull" factors that needs to be refined further. This could entail seeking out teens who stayed in school to ascertain if gender differences in these stressors hold and if their intensity is less (hence they had stayed in school). Theoretical sampling can also involve seeking out new types of data and re-interviewing study participants with new questions.

At this stage of analysis, researchers may turn to *schemas* to display categories and relationships. Strauss and Corbin (1994) offer a template schema that includes identifying *conditions, actions,* and *consequences.* As an example, this schema could be applied to an understanding of why homeless mentally ill clients "go AWOL" from residential programs, including the conditions or circumstances surrounding this act (rule-breaking, relapsing into drug abuse, etc.), the specifics of carrying it out (when, where, with whom, etc.), and the consequences that ensue (e.g., return to the streets or shelters).

Metaphors and *analogies* are frequently drafted into service (Lakoff & Johnson, 1980; Ryan & Bernard, 2003). The example of "going AWOL" illustrates the use of an analogy in coding in the NYSS. It was also an in vivo code, its origins in military usage obscured and broadened to include a variety of conditions surrounding the sudden departure from homeless residential programs. Metaphors can be invoked by the researcher or emerge in vivo. In the Harlem Mammogram Study in which I was involved, some of the women with breast cancer used a metaphor of gardening to describe how cancerous tumors took root and spread, one even saying, "I had a garden growing in there."

Bohm (2004, p. 273) adapted the work of Barney Glaser to describe several useful ways to approach qualitative data, including

1. Process (phases, transitions, sequences)
2. Degree or intensity
3. Typologies
4. Strategies (tactics, techniques, mechanisms)
5. Interactions (mutual effects, interdependence)
6. Identity (self-concept, self-reflection)
7. Turning points (critical junctures, point of no return)
8. Cultural and social norms
9. Consensus (conformity versus conflict)

These organizing frames constitute a set of options that a researcher may draw on—they are especially useful for graduate students and others new to qualitative methods.

To allow for a consistent frame of reference that transcends grounded theory, we will henceforth use the terms "themes" and "subthemes" to describe the culminating phases of data analysis. Themes take shape as the linkages between codes are mapped out, their ultimate value dependent on return passes through the data. Patton (2002) advises looking for recurring regularities or convergences in the data and ensuring that the emergent themes have internal homogeneity (all data indexed by them dovetail closely) and clear boundaries (minimal or no overlap across categories). Ideally, the full set of themes (and subthemes) captures all salient information.

Harking back to the earlier discussion of data displays suggested by Miles and Huberman (1994), some qualitative researchers construct a pyramid-type chart displaying subcodes at the bottom level, then codes, then code clusters or focused codes, and then categories or themes at the top. Others prefer to display the themes and subthemes as nodes and networks with linkages in between. (See Figure 8.2 for an example.) Researchers who wish to go the distance and develop a grounded theory are obliged to pursue the more demanding steps of testing their model and ensuring that all connections cohere into an integrated model.

Figure 8.2   Themes and Subthemes From Phase 1 of the NYSS

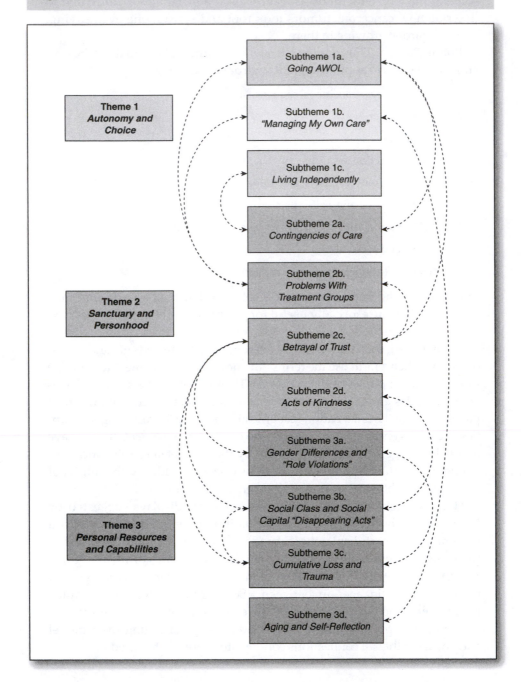

Keep in mind that field notes, interviewer observations, documents, and material items, in addition to transcripts, can be fodder for the analyst. Some of these can be coded directly while others are folded into analytic memos, their value distilled by the discerning researcher.

Beyond Coding

As important as it is, coding is only the starting point. Wider frames of reference can be employed (e.g., examining what participants do not talk about, whether intentionally or not; Bogdan & Taylor, 1975; Levy & Hollan, 2000). In Phase 1 of the NYSS, participants were asked to tell their life stories however they saw fit. Given their diagnosis of a major mental disorder, the literature led us to expect that this would figure prominently in their narratives. For the most part, however, this did not happen. Indeed, participants focused on their family troubles, the hardships of being homeless, problems with the law, and struggles with substance abuse. Mental illness was talked about, but most often in the context of unhappy treatment experiences and medication side effects (Padgett, Henwood, Abrams, & Davis, 2008).

One can also attend to form as well as content. In what can resemble (or eventually become) narrative analysis, the researcher may identify stories embedded in the text and note the meaning-making they imply. He may also take note of interesting vocabulary usage or paralinguistic phenomena such as long sighs, a quavering voice, or a hostile demeanor.

Here is an example of interacting with the data in a non-coding metaphoric way. While reading transcripts in the NYSS, we took note of the fact that men frequently referred to women as "females," as in "I would like to have a relationship with a female" or "Females have been a problem for me." This term of reference, common in street lingo, was not surprising to hear, but its frequency of use was noteworthy. Moreover, it appeared to fit with other evidence that a gender divide characterized participants' life experiences. Summarized in the interpretive phrase "outlaws versus outcasts," this divide cast homeless mentally ill women in gendered roles of victims—of physical and sexual assault, of sex trading, of pimps—and de-feminized outcasts, castigated as neglectful mothers. Their struggle for survival, a testimony to their resilience, was similar to that of their male counterparts but with this additional form of gendered adversity. Men, in contrast, could be "outlaws" (drug dealers, pimps, illegal vendors, absentee fathers) in masculine roles that gave them a measure of respect on the street (Padgett et al., 2006).

Multitasking During Coding: An Example From the NYSS

Box 8.5 shows an excerpt of an NYSS interview with a 32-year-old Latino man. (Some facts were changed to protect his identity.) Typical of many such interviews, there are several things going on here, some of them understood only by referring to the larger context of his life as well as what is known about drug addiction, parolee status, and so on. Javier (a pseudonym) is talking about getting out of prison and returning to his old neighborhood. He also mentions an earlier incident that ensued when he had an argument with his father and stormed out of his parents' apartment. On the street, he witnessed a mugging, stepped in to help the crime victim, and was attacked and sustained a serious head wound. Woven into this narrative are brief sidebars where Javier talks about his life and his struggle with drug addiction.

Box 8.5   An Interview Excerpt From the NYSS

144A: And, anyway I came out and I went back to the same neighborhood but I felt, "You know what, I can't stay in this house no more."

Interviewer: What neighborhood was that?

144A: A hundred fiftieth and Broadway, and uh, because that's where my people, places and things is at. All I have to do is show my face out in the front and they're already giving me stuff. And I said, "Then this'll you know, make it look bad for my PO [parole officer] if she finds out I got arrested again 'cause I wanted to get high." You know when I was getting high it was to, to block away the, the flashbacks of my violent past. And um, you know sometimes I would, you know, I asked God, "Why, why do I have to go through all of this? Um, what's the reason and purpose for it?" You know, now I'm, I'm learning to deal and accept I'm gonna die pretty soon.

Interviewer: Why do you believe that?

144A: See, when that young individual hit me over the head with a baseball bat, he didn't do it once, but 24 times. As you can see, my hair's starting to fall out in this section [gestures to his scalp]. . . . I'm willing to accept death. It happens. You know, I shouldn't have gotten into an argument with my father that day. But I'm going to college and this guy's [SP's father] stressing me out. So I decided to leave the house and I witnessed you know, a crime and um, it was, the reason why I got involved because the female [mugging victim] was six months pregnant. I'm the innocent bystander that got attacked.

Interviewer: When was that?

144A: That happened in 1998, yeah, 1998. Uh, I think about a, a, a yeah, a month after my birthday which I didn't celebrate either. And um, that's why life has been very difficult for me. You know and I, I keep trying, you know. Thank god I've got a work history you know, that I'm not making stuff up. I've really gone well beyond myself. . . . Because in my mind I'm going through my mid-life crisis and what, what's gonna be happening when I'm forty, fifty years old? Do I have to go through more difficulties?

The reader is invited to go to the exercises at the end of this chapter to practice open coding on this excerpt and also see how we ended up coding it. At the same time, even this small chunk of text offers several opportunities to interact with textual data in addition to coding. Here are a few general suggestions for going about this: (1) Write thoughts and observations in the left-hand margin; (2) flag information that is factual—in the NYSS, we use the letter "C" in the left margin to indicate this is a factual item that belongs in the individual's case summary; and (3) highlight exemplar quotes that might come in handy later—color-coded markers can be used to highlight these excerpts. Case summary information can also be code-worthy. Take, for example, a quote such as, "When my husband died in an auto accident, that was the end of the line for me." First, it indicates a "fact" of spousal death, and second, it chronicles the profound emotional impact of that event.

Returning to Javier's interview excerpt, we might note a few case summary items, for example, the date and circumstances of his brutal attack and the neighborhood where his drug problems originated. Using Strauss and Corbin's (1990) typology (mentioned earlier in this chapter), such "notes to self" might include the following:

1. Code note: Is the 12-step lingo of "people, places, and things" an in vivo code?

2. Theory notes: Javier attributes his drug abuse to earlier traumas—is this becoming a pattern in the sample? What does he mean by "I'm gonna die soon"? Is impending mortality a constant in SPs' lives? Is his worry about getting older part of a larger pattern in which SPs' awareness of advancing age and mortality push them toward recovery from substance abuse?

3. Operational notes:

Am I (interviewer) probing enough?
Check psychosocial records (from referring program) on when his parole ends.
Make sure incentive is sent to his mother as he requested.

These represent a small fraction of the queries, leads, and self-reflections that emerge when interacting with rich data. Staying close to the data is necessary but not sufficient. One must simultaneously frame one's observations within a larger context—whether that means constant comparisons with other interviews or with existing knowledge of the subject matter. As shown in Box 8.6, a code may have both meaning within a particular context and wider applications that "link up" to theories that were not part of the study's original conceptual framework.

Box 8.6	The Life of a Hardworking Code: Linking "Up and Out" to Theory

"Living independently" became a workhorse of a code in the NYSS, ultimately becoming a subtheme. (See Figure 8.2 on page 184.) Alternative code labels such as "need for housing" or "desire for autonomy" might have sufficed, but they did not do justice to participants' descriptions of what it was like to have their own apartment—either in the present or in a hoped-for future. Examining the many coded excerpts filed under "living independently" revealed more than just material comforts being invoked (or sought). Women talked about no longer needing to trade sex for shelter and being able to avoid abusive male friends. Men spoke of the freedom of being able to lock their door and of having clean clothing every day. Men and women alike noted the relief of not being under constant surveillance and supervision. These psychological benefits extended beyond the apartment walls, as participants noted how gratifying it felt to go out and know they had a safe place to return where they could cook their meals, watch television, entertain friends, or just be alone. Glaser (2002) writes about the staying power of concepts and their capacity to link a study's findings "up and out" to larger issues and ideas. Attempting to better understand what "living independently" meant in the context of housing status, I searched the public health and urban planning literature and came across the theory of ontological security. This produced a classic "aha" moment. R. D. Laing (1965) wrote that ontological insecurity was a problem for persons with schizophrenia whose mental illness deprived them of stable functioning and identity development. Sociologist Anthony Giddens (1990) developed a broad theory of ontological security for the postmodern era, arguing that many persons need (but lack) the constancy in their social and material environment that engenders self-actualization and faith in one's future. Interestingly, the literature revealed that empirical research on ontological security was largely confined to studies of home ownership (versus renting) in New Zealand and the United Kingdom. In this context, the leap from sleeping on a park bench to one's own apartment seemed especially momentous. Dupuis and Thorns's (1998) markers of ontological security related to having a home provided sensitizing concepts for me to use as I returned to the NYSS Phase 1 data to re-code and reanalyze. These markers included constancy, day-to-day routines, a sense of control due to a lack of surveillance, and a secure base from which identities can be constructed. These markers mapped onto the data beautifully. Moreover, as often happens, a new code emerged inductively from the analysis. Labeled "what's next," this code captured the anxiety felt by participants who had left behind the urgency of survival to face an uncertain future amidst the cumulative disability brought on by poverty, mental illness, and social exclusion (Padgett, 2007).

Commentary: This story of a code that proved to have deep interpretive traction exemplifies how "outside" theories may be brought into the study to help illuminate and refract meaning from the data. In this instance, it also shows how the outside theory can itself benefit from the association and gain broader explanatory power. Although most codes do not have this power, vigilance is needed to discriminate the leaders from the rank-and-file.

Using Qualitative Data Analysis (QDA) Software Part II: Facilitating Data Analysis

All QDA programs enable the researcher to code-and-retrieve (i.e., divide the text into coded chunks, attach codes to the chunks, and search and display these coded chunks on demand; Weitzman & Miles, 1995). Memos can be registered and linked to sections of data. In recent expansions of capacity, QDA software can handle non-text data (images, audio, and video) and insert hyperlinks to connect instantly to other files or data sources. Photographs can be coded in a similar manner (with portions blocked off and linked to a code label). Most programs provide ways to link codes into groups, in vertical hierarchies and schematic maps (a group of codes shown with linkages between them). Two-way frequency tables can be generated and uploaded into Microsoft Excel or statistical software for further analysis. Innovations in the newest versions include the ability to work with pdf files and Google Earth maps, transcribe audio files, work with spreadsheets, and use color coding and non-Roman text (e.g., Chinese characters).

Yet each program has its idiosyncratic terms—codes are "nodes" in NVivo and projects are "hermeneutic units" in ATLAS.ti—and each has quirks. Given the rapid pace of upgrades and increases in versatility, there will no doubt be additional features by the time you read this.

Coding on-screen is made easier by using a drop-down menu displaying the codebook and by the software's capacity to handle multiple overlapping coded sections. Auto-coding (text searching for code words) and "key word in context" (KWIC) searches can easily be performed, similar to using the "find" command in word processing. In the NYSS, we used ATLAS.ti to search for all versions of the word "help" (the wildcard designation allowing recognition of multiple forms such as *helped, helping,* etc.) on an initial pass through the data. This type of searching yields hits as well as misses, and the researcher must scrutinize the results to weed out the latter. Indeed, auto-coding and KWIC should not be confused with grounded theory and other types of meaning-centered analysis.

Filters and code selection commands are used to identify subsets of the data for further analysis and comparison. In addition to filtering by code label, one can select subsets of data according to characteristics such as sex, age, and the like. For example, men and women might be compared in their responses coded under "risky sexual experiences." Another useful function is the ability to create concept maps and plot horizontal or vertical connections between the nodes (e.g., "diet" and "exercise" can be connected to the higher-order code "self care"). These flexible network-making functions can display static relationships as well as flowcharts. Among the types of software, NVivo is oriented toward the creation of hierarchical tree structures, which is a better fit for some studies than others (Shiellerup, 2008).

QDA software programs are not inexpensive, and their site-licensing arrangements can be onerous (student discounts, on the other hand, are significant). As mentioned earlier, the software is worth the cost and effort if the researcher plans on using qualitative methods in the future or the study entails large amounts of data. All of the programs offer free introductory versions on their websites (see list at end of this chapter), and the reader is invited to try them out before making a purchase. The popularity of QDA software has raised concerns about the potential for over-structuring and mechanizing analyses and casting a misleading gloss of technological precision over what is always an untidy, iterative, and painstaking process. QDA software facilitates analysis, but it does not analyze the data. Indeed, computerized analyses do not offer the panoramic views of diverse forms of data that pre–computer era researchers cherish. Spreading out one's data on a large table (or the floor) allows the "simultaneous visual access to materials that makes ideas happen" (Agar, 1991, p. 193).

Using Numbers and Quantification in Qualitative Data Analyses

As mentioned earlier in this book, numbers may crop up during qualitative data analyses. Development of a typology, for example, could lead to reporting the number of participants associated with each type. According to Miles and Huberman (1994), counting themes via frequencies and percentages can help in identifying patterns or in verifying a hypothesis. At the same time, numbers and quantification must be approached carefully to avoid misleading the reader. Reporting the frequency of something, for example, can imply that a denominator exists when it does not. To state that 15 out of 20 adolescents mentioned going on drinking binges implies a "75% rate" of alcohol abuse, but this is only accurate if every teen was asked about drinking. Even if this sort of thing were done routinely, a rate calculated from such a small number of individuals has little import (and could be misunderstood if taken out of context). As noted by Morse (2007a), qualitative research favors describing "what is" rather than "how much."

Negative Case Analysis and Causation

In qualitative data analysis, the search for negative cases roughly corresponds to the quantitative researcher's reliance on a null hypothesis. In both instances, provisional theories are tested by searching for falsifying evidence (i.e., we become our own devil's advocate). This follows the logic of philosopher Karl Popper that hypotheses are not truly verified, but only supported in the absence of refuting evidence. As Albert Einstein said, "No amount of evidence can prove me right, and any amount of evidence can prove me wrong" (quoted in Miles & Huberman, 1994, p. 242).

Here is an example of how negative case analysis might be used. Let us say that you are interviewing overweight women and detect a pattern of childhood sexual abuse in their life stories. This leads you to theorize that childhood abuse is a contributor to overeating in adulthood. At this point, you are obligated to return to the data to search for negative cases—overweight women who did not experience childhood sexual abuse. Finding a disconfirming case need not lead you to completely discard the theory, but it does require serious reconsideration and caution. If the countervailing evidence becomes strong (i.e., negative cases start to pile up), it is time to let the theory go.

It is important to distinguish between *disconfirming evidence* (cases that refute an emerging theory) and *discrepant evidence* (cases that refine an emerging theory; Goetz & LeCompte, 1984). In the first instance, the exceptional case disallows the rule. In the second instance, it proves the rule but also refines and expands it.

The line between disconfirming and discrepant cases is blurry at times (Ely et al., 1991). Theories may become so refined and spread so thin that their explanatory value begins to sag under the weight of the evidence. A researcher may also be so taken with negative case analysis that she disconfirms every theme and achieves the dreaded state of analytic paralysis. Somewhere there is a happy medium—a mixture of enthusiasm tempered by skepticism. In the meantime, it is probably better to err on the side of caution than to throw it to the wind.

Where does this leave qualitative researchers when questions of causation arise? Experts run the gamut of opinions about this, ranging from relative enthusiasm (Miles & Huberman, 1994) to serious doubt (Lofland & Lofland, 1995). On the sidelines, anti-positivist skeptics question whether the search for causation is plausible or desirable, given the postmodern premise that facts are "fictitious" (Lofland & Lofland, 1995). As with so many contested issues in qualitative research, one's position depends in large part on one's epistemological stance.

Secondary Analysis and Meta-Synthesis

Given the sizeable investments of time and resources that go into a qualitative study, it makes sense that researchers are increasingly willing to share their data with others. Secondary analyses extend the life of a study and are an efficient use of resources. As a general rule, richer and more complex data offer more fertile ground for secondary analyses than narrow or thin data. In the NYSS, the Phase 1 life history data have turned out to be a mother lode open to "mining" from different perspectives and with different methods of analysis. The Phase 2 interviews follow specific domains and are more circumscribed, thus narrowing analytic options.

Secondary analyses may be carried out by the original research team, by some of its members in collaboration with new researchers, or by an entirely new investigative team with minimal knowledge of the original study. Regardless of who is involved, there is the potential problem of retrofitting new research questions to the earlier data (Van den Berg, 2005; Williams & Collins, 2002). Qualitative data have undergone their own filtering and sorting processes unknown to subsequent investigators. The norms for maintaining audit trails are far from agreed on within qualitative research, and many investigators either avoid doing so or reject it on the principle that it is too constraining. Finally, the immersion and interconnectedness of researcher and participant, one of the most rewarding and informing aspects of qualitative research, are missing from secondary analyses. Qualitative researchers who prefer collaborative models of inquiry with their study participants would find this unsatisfying.

On the positive side, gaining institutional review board approval for secondary analyses is usually much easier because interacting with "human subjects" is not involved. Yet secondary analyses are not without ethical risks. Identifying information, for example, can inhere in the data even when the names of participants are not included (Thorne, 1998). The respect for privacy and awareness of context that characterized earlier relationships may be missing on the second go-round. Data from a study of abortion among college students, for example, could become the basis for interpretations that range well beyond what the study participants believe they had signed on for in the first place.

Meta-syntheses involve aggregating the findings from several qualitative studies of the same topic to draw conclusions for comparative purposes (Dixon-Woods & Fitzpatrick, 2001). Like their quantitative counterpart (meta-analysis), qualitative meta-syntheses have been touted as essential for identifying evidence-based practices (Pope, Mays, & Popay, 2007; Thorne, Jensen, Kearny, Noblit, & Sandelowski, 2004). Thus, the pursuit of "what works" in evidence-based practice can be enhanced by examining "what is at work" when individuals and communities experience interventions and report these experiences in their own words (Saini & Shlonsky, 2011).

Not surprisingly, qualitative meta-syntheses present epistemological and methodological challenges arising from the lack of uniformity in methods as well as in the terminology used to report these methods. The idiosyncratic and nonspecific features of many qualitative studies can produce "apples and oranges" problems poorly suited to aggregation. There is also the potential for overlooking or even intensifying biases present in a group of studies being synthesized. For example, most qualitative studies of persons with schizophrenia have relied heavily or exclusively on white or Caucasian respondents, even though African Americans are disproportionately diagnosed with the illness. Synthesizing findings from these samples will almost certainly misrepresent the experience of schizophrenia.

Despite these limitations, meta-syntheses of qualitative studies are necessary for knowledge development. Otherwise, their findings are missing from what is already a meta-analytic movement steeped in quantification and randomized trials (Pope et al., 2007). While the challenges will not be easily resolved, the benefits in terms of representation are considerable.

Hybrid and Mixed Qualitative Approaches to Data Analysis

As discussed in Chapter 2, researchers often choose to mix and match qualitative approaches. This can occur at different stages of a study and unfold in differing combinations and for different purposes. It can also introduce problems in the form of method and data incongruities (Johnstone, 2004; Wimpenny & Gass, 2000). As noted by Annells (2006), mixing at the analytic level can be problematic if the underlying philosophical paradigms are in conflict—a lesser concern for pragmatists.

Arguing in favor of hybrid vigor, Fereday and Muir-Cochrane (2006) used inductive and deductive thematic analyses by mixing Boyatzis's (1998) inductive methods with Crabtree and Miller's (1999) template style of coding to study nurses in their day-to-day performance. Thus, data-driven codes from participant interviews, such as "trust and respect," were combined with theory-driven codes, for example, "reciprocity," to produce an integrated model of performance feedback and self-assessment in nursing practice. Uehara (2001) creatively blended narrative analysis with event structure analysis (Griffin, 1993) to trace the temporal sequencing of events as a Cambodian American family sought help for the "spirit invasion" experienced by their severely distressed mother.

An example of sequential use can be found in Beck's (1993) study of postpartum depression in which she conducted phenomenological analyses followed by grounded theory analyses of the data. Close concordance was found between the two sets of findings, thus lending credence to her development of a substantive theory explaining the onset and course of depression shortly after the birth of a child. Agar and MacDonald (1995) used juxtaposition to compare the results of conversation analyses of focus group data (in which teens discussed drug abuse) with their ethnographic observations of adolescent drug use.

Saturation and Interpretation

Interpretation deals with the less obvious and more abstract dimensions of the data, the act of "reading into" and "extracting meaning from." All research involves interpretation, whether of numbers or narrative; quantitative studies tend to be restrained and cautious, letting the statistical findings tell most of the story. In contrast, qualitative studies operate from a premise of greater interpretive latitude, their ultimate contribution dependent on how this latitude is handled. Multidisciplinary perspectives are especially helpful in this phase because they offer diverse ideas and framing devices for understanding what is going on.

The concept of *saturation* in this context refers to the point at which no additional data collection is needed, no new codes are developed, and themes and subthemes have been fully fleshed out (Bowen, 2008; Morse, 1995). Originating in grounded theory, saturation has been adopted by a variety of qualitative approaches as an answer to the inevitable question, how much is enough? Studies with modest aims and a priori codes are likely to be saturated much sooner than more ambitious and inductive endeavors.

Saturation does not depend on word or incident counts and frequencies because fullness comes from depth rather than breadth. Perhaps not surprisingly, it is easier to assert having reached this stage than to prove it (Morse, 1995), although careful documentation and memo writing can alleviate some concerns about premature closure. The alternatives to saturation—an endpoint set in advance or a decision based on arbitrary criteria—are a poor fit for qualitative inquiry. Box 8.7 offers a rare case example documenting how saturation is achieved and ends with a cautionary note.

Box 8.7   Operationalizing Saturation: A Study of Sex Workers in West Africa

Guest, Bunce, and Johnson (2006) decided to explore the question of saturation empirically using data analyses from their qualitative study of sex workers in West Africa. When, they asked, would the codebook be complete and no further changes needed? Would 6 interviews yield as much information as 12, 30, or 60 interviews? Could coding activity slow down to a trickle after X number of interviews, and then suddenly yield new codes much later after "saturation" had presumably been achieved? Starting with 60 interviews, they began coding in increments of 6, keeping track of the number of codes and code definitions as they proceeded. Here is what they found:

- After coding the first 30 interviews, the codebook contained 109 codes of which 80 (73%) were identified within the first six transcripts.
- Of the remaining 29 codes, 20 were identified in transcripts 6–12 (now up to 90% of all codes).
- Coding of transcripts 31–60 yielded only five new codes; four of these were spin-offs from existing codes rather than entirely new information.
- The strength or reach of a code was measured by the number of interviews in which it occurred rather than the number of coded excerpts (because talkative interviewees could easily skew the data).

Of the 36 high-frequency codes, 34 had been identified within the first six transcripts. Guest and colleagues concluded that 12 interviews would have been sufficient (rather than the 60 they conducted). However, they offered a few caveats about this finding. First, they used a standardized list of open-ended questions about beliefs and experiences surrounding sex work. Studies with more improvisational questioning would not be likely to yield such a stable list of codes early on. Second, the coders had similar backgrounds and knowledge about the phenomenon so that consensus—even when coding independently—was probably easier. Finally, their sample was relatively homogeneous. Response variation led more often to definitional tweaking than to coding overhauls (dropping codes, adding new ones, etc.).

Commentary: Qualitative researchers naturally fear that premature closure of data collection will deprive them of vital information waiting just around the corner. Yet unnecessary interviews and diminishing returns drain scarce resources and burden respondents. The study done by Guest and colleagues is innovative for taking on the "saturation threshold" as an empirical question. Yet its findings cannot be generalized too far because they were based on several restrictive premises that do not fit most qualitative studies.

Interpretation gains momentum as the analysis proceeds; memos log this process but also propel it forward. Meaning comes from the linkages or interstices as well as the building blocks that comprise the themes and subthemes (Miles & Huberman, 1994). These relationships may be temporal (as in stages and phases) or, more commonly, conceptual networks arrayed in horizontal or vertical (hierarchical) fashion. Searching for disconfirming cases, serendipitous relationships, and paradoxes helps open up the process and keep it fresh.

Interpretation brings in the larger context (i.e., applying interpretive frames from the literature and from the realms of practice and policy). Having thorough knowledge of related research lends greater sophistication as well as wider applicability. Are the findings consistent with this literature? Do they expand on what is already known? Do they challenge the received wisdom? Qualitative research has a unique capacity for debunking the status quo. Elliot Liebow's classic work *Talley's Corner* (1967) has endured because it forced a reconsideration of stereotypes about the lives of African American men in the 1960s.

An Example of a Conceptual Schema

Figure 8.2 (on page 184) shows the conceptual model developed from Phase 1 of the NYSS. The model has a visual and schematic logic, but narrative description is needed to make it come to life. Although space limitations preclude full elaboration, certain features can be pointed out to illustrate thematic development. As shown, the three themes are autonomy and choice (Theme 1), sanctuary and personhood (Theme 2), and personal resources and capabilities (Theme 3). The subthemes elaborate on each theme and comprise its full content (subthemes 1a and 1b were in vivo codes).

The dotted arrows show connections among the subthemes. The longest dotted arrow, for example, shows that participants desire to "manage their own care" (subtheme 1b)—as in fiddling with medication dosages and quitting drug abuse without treatment—was associated with reflections on advancing age and the need to take charge of their lives (subtheme 3d).

The model's theoretical uplinks are noteworthy. As described in Box 8.6 on pages 188–189, the code "living independently" graduated to become a subtheme that aligned with the theory of ontological security (and expanded the theory beyond its original scope). Themes 1 and 2 in the model are emic, that is, rooted in participants' perspectives. Theme 3, on the other hand, is etic in that it captures our observations filtered through social science theories and ideas. All of the subthemes under Theme 3 had enough empirical and conceptual salience to support separate analyses and manuscripts for publication. These include subthemes 3a and 3c on gender and trauma (Padgett et al., 2006), subtheme 3b on social network depletion (Hawkins & Abrams, 2007), and subtheme 3d on the effects of aging and self-reflection (Shibusawa & Padgett, 2009). Theories and concepts found applicable to the data and analyses included feminist, trauma, and social capital theories as well as the life course perspective.

In Pursuit of Methodological Transparency

Qualitative reports often obscure full description of their methods. This state of affairs reflects a tradition of eliding methodological description in the absence of agreed-on procedures. This, in turn, leaves novice researchers struggling to emulate their role models from afar with inadequate instruction.

This chapter represents a modest attempt to redress this situation and to join forces with qualitative researchers who have similar commitments to transparency (Charmaz's 2006 book on grounded theory being one example). Demystifying qualitative methods makes them more accessible, and it facilitates cross-disciplinary communication (Ryan & Bernard, 2003). To be sure, an overemphasis on documentation can lead to superficiality and dampen creativity. Yet a study's findings and conclusions inspire much greater confidence when built on methodological transparency.

Summary and Concluding Thoughts

This chapter began by offering guidelines for managing and analyzing data and strengthening the development of conceptual schemas via negative case analysis, theoretical sampling, and other strategies. Computer software facilitates these activities in a number of helpful ways, but it does not actually analyze the data.

Despite a dizzying array of possibilities, most qualitative data analyses have the following in common: (1) full and repeated immersions in the data, (2) going "deep" into descriptive specificity as well as "across" with pattern recognition, (3) attending to context—temporal and environmental, and (4) proceeding "up and out" to weave in theoretical and empirical knowledge from the literature. Analysis begins inductively, but the pathways to its completion often include deductive thinking as well. The insider perspective is an invaluable part of this process, but the ultimate contribution of a qualitative study depends on the probity and intellectual clarity of its interpretations.

Each of the six qualitative approaches has its own analytic traditions, but the emphasis in this chapter was given to what is done most often (i.e., coding and thematic development). Whether this leads to a fully developed grounded theory or, more commonly, an interpretive framework, such analytic involvement is an exercise in restraint (from becoming weighed down by a priori ideas and concepts) and creativity (comparing and contrasting, searching for what is unusual and unknown).

Despite its demands, qualitative data analysis is exciting, a necessary step to making previous efforts come to fruition. The sense of accomplishment—of producing new knowledge—can be immensely gratifying. Candid and thorough description of methods goes a long way toward making them accessible. And for those seeking mastery on their own, three words come to mind: practice, practice, practice.

EXERCISES

1. Instructors who have transcripts of qualitative interviews can share portions with their students and ask them to code the interviews. Students then meet in groups and discuss their codes and the reasoning behind them.

2. In the classroom, students focus on a common experience (such as their reasons for going to graduate school) and break up into small groups to discuss the topic and expand on it as much as possible. Next, refer to Bohm's (2004) nine organizing frames listed earlier in this chapter and choose one or two as a way to think about these experiences. Have each group discuss their "findings," stating whether they took the form of a typology, sequencing, and so on.

3. Read the excerpt in Box 8.5 and choose one of the following options to analyze it:

Option A: Open code the text (using line numbers to show what segments go with what code). Discuss your codes with a colleague who has independently open-coded the same excerpt.

Option B: Take a look at the list of NYSS codes below and assign them to the text as you see fit. (Use line numbers to identify the segments that go with each code.) Note that the code abbreviation is followed by its full label or title and its definition in parentheses.

NE—refers to "neighborhood effects" (can be negative or positive, for example, drug temptations and crime dangers as well as feelings of support from neighbors and local community)

SA/U—"substance abuse/use talk" (when SP talks about drinking and illicit drug use)

SR/LP—"self-reflection/life perspectives" (reflections on one's life; includes what went right and what went wrong)

VIO/VIC—"violence and victimization" (episodes of being violently attacked or otherwise victimized; also includes perpetration of violence)

The following are suggested "answers" for Option B. Keep in mind that these are not hard and fast—coding decisions are rarely uniform. Your answers may vary somewhat, but the central meaning or idea of the code should be present in each excerpt so labeled.

NE (lines 2–9); SA/U (lines 2–11); VIO/VIC (lines 16–28); SR/LP (lines 9–14 and 27–32)

Additional Readings

Bernard, H. R. (Ed.). (2000). *Handbook of methods in cultural anthropology.* Walnut Creek, CA: AltaMira Press.

Charmaz, C. (2006). *Constructing grounded theory: A practical guide through qualitative analysis.* Thousand Oaks, CA: Sage.

Coffey, A., & Atkinson, P. (1996). *Making sense of qualitative data.* Thousand Oaks, CA: Sage.

Corbin, J., & Strauss, A. L. (2008). *Basics of qualitative research* (3rd ed.). Thousand Oaks, CA: Sage.

Dey, I. (1993). *Qualitative data analysis: A user-friendly guide for social scientists.* New York: Routledge.

Dey, I. (1999). *Grounding grounded theory: Guidelines for qualitative inquiry.* San Diego, CA: Academic Press.

Gee, J. P. (2005). *An introduction to discourse analysis: Theory and method.* London: Routledge.

Hsieh, H., & Shannon, S. E. (2005). Three approaches to qualitative content analysis. *Qualitative Health Research, 15*(9), 1277–1288.

Krippendorf, K. (2004). *Content analysis: An introduction to its methodology* (2nd ed.). Thousand Oaks, CA: Sage.

LeCompte, M. D., & Schensul, J. J. (2010). *Designing and conducting ethnographic research* (2nd ed.). (*Ethnographer's Toolkit,* Vol. 1). Walnut Creek, CA: AltaMira Press.

Lofland, J., & Lofland, L. (1995). *Analyzing social settings: A guide to qualitative observation and analysis* (3rd ed.). Belmont, CA: Wadsworth.

Miles, M. B., & Huberman, A. M. (1994). *Qualitative data analysis* (2nd ed.). Thousand Oaks, CA: Sage.

Moustakas, C. (1994). *Phenomenological research methods.* Thousand Oaks, CA: Sage.

Patton, M. Q. (2002). *Qualitative research and evaluation methods* (3rd ed.). Thousand Oaks, CA: Sage.

Riessman, C. (1993). *Narrative analysis.* Newbury Park, CA: Sage.

Saini, M., & Shlonsky, A. (2011). *Systematic syntheses of qualitative research.* New York: Oxford University Press.

Saldana, J. (2009). *The coding manual for qualitative researchers.* Thousand Oaks, CA: Sage.

Smith, C., & Short, P. M. (2001). Integrating technology to improve the efficiency of qualitative data analysis: A note on methods. *Qualitative Sociology, 24*(3), 401–407.

Stake, R.E. (2005). *Multiple case study analysis.* Thousand Oaks, CA: Sage.

Tesch, R. (1990). *Qualitative research: Analysis types and software tools.* Philadelphia, PA: Falmer Press.

Thorne, S. (2000). Data analysis in qualitative research. *Evidence-Based Nursing, 3,* 68–70.

Weston, C., Gambell, T., Beauchamp, J., McAlpine, N., Wiseman, C., & Beauchamp, C. (2001). Analyzing interview data: The development and evolution of a coding system. *Qualitative Sociology, 24*(3), 381–400.

Yin, R. K. (2008). *Case study research: Design and methods* (4th ed.). Thousand Oaks, CA: Sage.

QDA Software Resources

Readings

Fielding, N., & Lee, R. (Eds.). (1998). *Computer analysis in qualitative research.* Thousand Oaks, CA: Sage.

Gibbs, G. R. (2007). Media review: ATLAS.ti software to assist in the qualitative analysis of data. *Journal of Mixed Methods Research, 1*(1), 103–104.

Kelle, U. (1996). *Computer-aided qualitative data analysis: Theory, methods, and practice.* Thousand Oaks, CA: Sage.

Lewins, A., & Silver, C. (2007). *Using software in qualitative research: A step-by-step guide.* London: Sage.

Lewis, R. B. (2004). NVivo 2.0 and ATLAS.ti 5.0: A comparative analysis of two popular qualitative data analysis programs. *Field Methods, 16,* 439–464.

Miles, M. B., & Weitzman, E. A. (1994). Choosing computer programs for qualitative data analysis. In M. B. Miles & A. M. Huberman (Eds.), *Qualitative data analysis: An expanded sourcebook* (2nd ed.). Thousand Oaks, CA: Sage.

Richard, L. (1999). Data alive! The thinking behind NVivo. *Qualitative Health Research, 9*(3), 88–93.

Richards, T. J., & Richards, L. (1994). Using computers in qualitative research. In N. K. Denzin & Y. S. Lincoln (Eds.), *Handbook of qualitative research* (pp. 445–462). Thousand Oaks, CA: Sage.

Weitzman, E., & Miles, M. (1995). *Computer programs for qualitative data analysis: A software sourcebook.* Thousand Oaks, CA: Sage.

Software Information

An excellent independent resource (not supported by a software company) can be found online at http://caqdas.soc.surrey.ac.uk

An overview of QDA software can be found at http://www.quarc.de/overview .html. Student discounts are available as long as proof of eligibility is offered.

Products

http://www.scolari.com (information and downloadable software demos for ATLAS.ti, NUD*IST, The Ethnograph, etc.

ATLAS.ti: http://www.atlasti.com

CDC EZ-Text (free download): http://www.cdc.gov/hiv/topics/surveillance/ resources/software/ez-text/index.htm

The Ethnograph: http://www.qualisresearch.com

HyperRESEARCH: http://www.researchware.com

NUD*IST: http://www.qsrinternational.com

NVivo: http://www.qsrinternational.com

9

Strategies for Rigor

One of the most vexing questions in qualitative research centers on defining what is "a good, valid, and/or trustworthy qualitative study" (Sandelowski & Barroso, 2002, p. 2). Glaser and Strauss addressed this question with a chapter on "The Credibility of Grounded Theory" in their 1967 seminal work, Lincoln and Guba (1985) provided their own discussions of quality, and others have followed suit (Bradley, Curry, & Devers, 2007; Inui & Frankel, 1991; Morrow, 2005; Padgett, 2008; Pope & Mays, 1995; Sandelowski & Barroso, 2002).

Perhaps not surprisingly, consensus on standards for quality has been elusive. Miles and Huberman (1994) wrote of this dilemma, "We have the unappealing double bind whereby qualitative studies can't be verified because researchers don't report on their methodology, and they don't report on their methodology because there are no established canons or conventions for doing so" (p. 244). Critics of qualitative methods are emboldened by this impasse. How, they ask, can one trust findings from studies where standards are shifting and subject to diverse interpretations?

The ever-changing landscape of qualitative inquiry virtually guarantees that opinions about rigor will differ, one of few areas of agreement being a rejection of traditional quantitative criteria (Altheide & Johnson, 1994; Whittemore, Chase, & Mandle, 2001). Pivotal to discussions about quality have been different ideas about the role of subjectivity, the stance of the researcher, and who has the authority and legitimacy to judge good versus bad qualitative research.

Subjectivity is an essential element of qualitative inquiry since the insider perspective is valued (Ellis & Flaherty, 1992). Once distance and objectivity cease to be operating principles, the researcher's subjectivity is also acknowledged and, to varying degrees, managed through *reflexivity*, or systematic self-awareness. Feminist researchers were among the first to break down traditional researcher–researched boundaries, promoting in their stead a close partnership (Fonow & Cook, 1991; Reinharz, 1992). Differing opinions about the optimal degree of researcher subjectivity often animate debates about what constitutes rigor. In this chapter, we will briefly review these debates, discuss some of the threats to trustworthiness in qualitative research, and end with recommendations for strategies to improve rigor.

Evaluating Qualitative Research: Debates About Standards and Strategies

Virtually all qualitative researchers reject the traditional quantitative standards of reliability and validity, but agreement usually stops there. To constructivists, a consensual set of criteria would raise the specter of intrusive oversight reminiscent of positivism. To pragmatists, standards of quality are needed, but the struggle to identify and agree on them can be a difficult (though worthwhile) effort.

A critical distinction arises at this point: Evidence of quality emerging from a completed study is not the same as building into a study's design deliberate efforts to improve quality. *Evaluative standards* are applied to *completed* studies; *strategies for rigor* are pursued *during* the study. Few (if any) qualitative researchers would argue against taking specific actions to ensure that a study is of high quality, but disagreements can arise over what those actions should be.

Evaluative Criteria and External Standards

Lincoln and Guba (1985) were in the vanguard when it came to developing separate criteria applicable to qualitative methods (which they initially called naturalistic inquiry). Drawing direct parallels from quantitative research, they proposed credibility, transferability, auditability, and confirmability as alternatives to internal validity, external validity, reliability, and objectivity. Together, these connoted the *trustworthiness* of a qualitative study.

Credibility is the degree of fit between respondents' views and the researcher's description and interpretations. *Transferability* refers to generalizability, not of the sample (as in quantitative terms) but of the study's findings. External validity is not a priority because the focus is on subjective meanings and depth over breadth (Donmoyer, 1990). *Auditability* (or *dependability*) means that the study's procedures are documented and traceable—they need not lead to the same conclusions but should have a logic that makes sense to others. *Confirmability* is achieved by demonstrating that the study's findings were not imagined or concocted but, rather, firmly linked to the data.

Lincoln and Guba's (1985) criteria did not receive universal acclaim or adoption, but they served an important purpose in offering alternatives to quantitative standards. Later, additional terms were offered such as *truthfulness* (instead of validity), *consistency* (instead of reliability; Slevin & Sines, 2000), and *reflexive accounting* (Altheide & Johnson, 1994). Others have turned to literary standards of rhetoric and persuasiveness or to the humanities where elegance, consistency, and coherence are emblematic of quality (McCracken, 1988).

The Meaning(s) of Generalizability in Qualitative Methods

Generalizability in qualitative research is subject to differing opinions. Constructivists have led the way in questioning its relevance, arguing that an emphasis on generalizing strips away the context that imbues a qualitative study with credibility. Ethnographies have been lauded for their intrinsic value—few would argue that Malinowski's (1922) classic studies of the Trobriand Islanders are deficient because they lack generalizability.

Much has changed in the world as well as in qualitative methods since the early 20th century. Qualitative studies can still have intrinsic interest, but this particular raison d'être has lost ground as expectations have been ramped up in academic as well as applied settings where findings are expected to have wider ramifications.

Maxwell (2002) defined *generalizability* as having different levels of meaning, one referring to extending one's findings from the sample to others in the setting who were not included in the study, and other levels referring to wider contexts for extrapolation. For example, can the findings from a study of youth gangs in Los Angeles be applied to local gang members who were not interviewed? What about youth gangs in Chicago, in Rio de Janeiro, or gangs in general? It is reasonable to inquire about these outwardly radiating circles of inference—sometimes referred to as *transferability*—because localized knowledge without larger meaning has questionable value.

Turning the tables, it is fair to say that generalizability is often a problem in quantitative studies because many are unable to meet the assumptions of random sampling, normal distributions, and bounded sampling frames that underlie inferential statistics. Sophisticated sampling and polling techniques have had better success at this, but large-scale surveys constitute a small part of the research agenda in public health. Most populations of interest—for example, abused women, substance abusers, immigrant families, and persons with AIDS—cannot be randomly sampled.

To their credit, the vast majority of qualitative researchers neither make extravagant claims nor try to "chew more than they bite off." Whether and how far qualitative findings can be extrapolated depends on what claims are being made. That qualitative studies do not share the inferential ambitions of quantitative research does not mean that they eschew applicability (or transferability) altogether. A qualitative evaluation of a malaria prevention program, for example, has far more impact if its results can be used to inform other malaria programs. Qualitative researchers desire fame (if not fortune) as much as anyone and know full well that the farther their findings resonate the better. Findings can have transferability and resonance without being "generalizable" in a statistical sense based on how the sample was selected. The capacity for a study to stimulate thought, improve practices and policies, and incite further research is a metric of success agreeable to most anyone.

Threats to the Trustworthiness of Qualitative Studies

Lincoln and Guba's (1985) concept of *trustworthiness* comes closest to capturing what is meant by rigor and accountability in qualitative research. A trustworthy study is one that is carried out fairly and ethically and whose findings represent as closely as possible the experiences of the respondents (Steinmetz, 1991). Trustworthiness is not a matter of blind faith; it must be demonstrated and earned.

Threats to trustworthiness fall under three broad headings: reactivity, researcher biases, and respondent biases. *Reactivity* refers to the potentially distorting effects of the researcher's presence on participants' beliefs and behaviors; the intensity and closeness of qualitative research relationships make this an obvious concern.

Researcher biases emerge when observations and interpretations are clouded by preconceptions and personal opinions of the researcher. Thus, investigators may choose informants who are simpatico with their worldview, may ask leading questions to get the answers they want, or may ignore data that do not support their conclusions. Emotional pitfalls can also contribute to researcher biases. The unwary qualitative researcher may veer too far in either direction—overly familiar or estranged—and thus lose his effectiveness.

Finally, there is the threat of *respondent bias.* This issue is a bit trickier to talk about because it implies that the respondents' subjectivity can sometimes be questioned. Respondents may withhold information and even lie to protect their privacy or to avoid revealing unpleasant truths. Inquiring about illegal drug use and sexual activity is likely to bring this about, but any topic can prompt a desire to conceal or mislead. At the other extreme, participants may try to be helpful and offer answers that they believe we (or the larger society) want to hear.

Rather than deliberately mislead, respondents may have faulty recall or interpret events in a way that conflicts with what the researcher "knows" from another source. What does one do, for example, if the clinic records say a pregnant woman has tested positive for HIV, yet she does not mention this during the interview? Getting at the "truth" may be worth risking a confrontation, but it is usually better left alone, at least until a more propitious time when rapport and trust have deepened. Focusing too literally on truthfulness can turn the researcher into an interrogator.

These three types of threats to trustworthiness—reactivity, researcher bias, and respondent bias—affect all studies, whether quantitative or qualitative. Although the intensity of the research relationship places qualitative studies in greater jeopardy with regard to the first two types of threats, such studies have an advantage with regard to the third (respondent biases). After all, faulty memory, concealment, or outright lying are less likely to occur in trusting, in-depth relationships.

Strategies for Rigor in Qualitative Research

Even when viewed favorably, qualitative methods are frequently misunderstood. I have encountered many friendly doubts voiced by researcher colleagues who wonder about small sample sizes and obtuse methods.

One way to help alleviate doubts is to offer a clear rationale for using qualitative methods (Marshall & Rossman, 2006; Morse, 1994; Munhall, 1994). While this may seem to be an unfair burden (quantitative researchers need not do this), it is in fact an opportunity to educate the reader and convey a sense of mastery. When the topic is appropriate, this is an easy argument to make.

In the following paragraphs, I will discuss six strategies for enhancing rigor and trustworthiness culled from the literature in qualitative research. Although not all are relevant or feasible for any given study, they represent an array of techniques intended to address one or more of the threats to trustworthiness described above.

Prolonged Engagement

Arising from the early days of anthropological fieldwork, prolonged engagement has come to be a defining characteristic of qualitative studies regardless of where they take place. As shown in Figure 9.1, prolonged engagement helps to ameliorate reactivity and respondent bias. Thus, the effects of the researcher's presence dissipate considerably when she spends long periods of time in the field and becomes accepted (or at least benignly tolerated).

Prolonged engagement makes withholding information or lying by respondents less likely. As Elliot Liebow (1993) noted, "lies do not really hold up well over long periods of time" (p. 321). An experienced researcher can often tell when respondents are shading the truth or lying, but it usually takes more than one encounter to do so. For interview-based studies, prolonged engagement may not be possible. (However, as discussed in Chapter 7, conducting more than one interview is a step toward accomplishing this goal.)

One drawback of prolonged engagement is the risk of researcher bias. Researchers can go too far in either direction—they can "go native" and lose all interpretive distance or experience the "familiarity breeds contempt" problem. Nevertheless, the advantages far outweigh the disadvantages.

Triangulation

The term *triangulation*, borrowed from navigational science and land surveying, originally referred to using two or more sources to achieve a comprehensive picture of a fixed point of reference. Four types of triangulation were outlined by Denzin (1978):

1. *Theory triangulation:* The use of multiple theories or perspectives to interpret a single set of data.

2. *Methodological triangulation:* The use of multiple methods to study a single topic.

3. *Observer triangulation:* The use of more than one observer in a single study to achieve intersubjective agreement.

4. *Data triangulation:* The use of more than one data source (interviews, archival materials, observational data, etc.).

Valerie Janesick (2000) added a fifth type of triangulation: *interdisciplinary triangulation,* or using more than one discipline in a single study.

From its earliest use as a means of confirmation, triangulation has expanded in definition to include *completeness* and the *enlargement of perspectives* (Flick, 2004). Triangulation by theory and triangulation by discipline are a good fit with this new definition. Triangulation by method most often refers to using qualitative and quantitative approaches in tandem. As discussed in Chapter 3, this can be done for confirmation or completeness depending on the study's purposes.

Having multiple coders could be considered a form of *analytic triangulation,* although the latter could be more broadly construed to include interpretations from different perspectives. As discussed in Chapter 8, independent coding and comparison are valuable safeguards against bias in data analysis. Triangulation by data source—the most common type—is typically used for corroboration or confirmation. When data from field notes, interviews, or archival materials are convergent, one has greater confidence that the observations are trustworthy. As shown in Figure 9.1, triangulation helps to counter all of the threats to trustworthiness. Yet, inconsistencies and contradictions are common (Bloor, 1997). When this happens, one must decide whether to favor one source over another or view discrepancies as an opportunity for new insights. Just as negative case analysis may open the door to refining one's interpretations, disagreement among data sources may lead to new and expanded perspectives.

Figure 9.1   Strategies for Enhancing Rigor and Trustworthiness

Threat to trustworthiness

Strategy	Reactivity	Researcher Bias	Respondent Bias
Prolonged Engagement	+	–	+
Triangulation	+	+	+
Peer Debriefing/ Support	0	+	0
Member Checking	+	+	+
Negative Case Analysis	0	+	0
Audit Trail	0	+	0

+	Positive effect in reducing threat
–	Negative effect in reducing threat
0	No effect

Peer Debriefing and Support

Debriefing and support often go unheralded as a means of keeping the "instrument" sharp and true. Such support often comes from an academic advisor or a mentor, but one of the most effective means is *peer debriefing and support* (PDS; Padgett, Mathew, & Conte, 2004). For qualitative studies conducted by a group rather than a solo investigator, the research team can become the de facto PDS group.

PDS groups can be a lifeline for qualitative researchers (Steinmetz, 1991). Members get and give feedback, offer fresh ideas, and simply recharge their batteries. Attending a PDS group meeting gives the researcher a chance to share the emotional ups and downs of fieldwork and data analysis. However, the role of these groups in qualitative research is not simply socio-emotional. They are also a mechanism for keeping the researcher honest (Lincoln & Guba, 1985). To this end, PDS groups contribute to the rigor of a qualitative study by reducing researcher bias (see Figure 9.1).

PDS group members may present ideas or hunches for feedback. They may share portions of their coding memos along with relevant chunks of data to see if the codes make sense. Group members may also share passages from their field notes and journals to get reactions from others about their observations and their ability to be self-reflexive. Some group members may become reciprocal co-coders. There are rarely any set rules as long as confidentiality is maintained and the focus stays on constructive criticism.

PDS groups work best when they meet on a regular schedule (monthly or bimonthly) and rotate leadership roles among group members. Their composition can be homogeneous by discipline or they may be multidisciplinary. Homogeneity allows members to draw on common interests, communicate in a common language, and reduce time spent negotiating disciplinary boundaries. Heterogeneous groups drawn from diverse fields can be intellectually invigorating. For qualitative researchers who do not have access to a PDS group, acquiring even one peer can be helpful.

In addition to their rigor-enhancing qualities, PDS groups perform instrumental functions. Group members give helpful hints, for example, remembering to take extra batteries to interviews. They share news of the latest in qualitative data analysis (QDA) software and tips on how to use it. They encourage each other to set and meet deadlines in completing the project. They might offer suggestions on how to negotiate with an unhappy spouse or partner who is feeling neglected due to the researcher's time spent in the field.

PDS groups have potential limitations as well. They can collectively veer off course, either by fostering a "groupthink" atmosphere of enforced conformity or by becoming hypercritical and intolerant. New ideas are fragile creations and can get crushed even by well-meaning colleagues (Wolcott, 2009). Second, their logistical requirements of scheduling and agenda setting can be daunting in this era of competing interests. However, when done properly, peer support is an invaluable addition to the repertoire of rigor enhancement.

Member Checking

Member checking (Lincoln & Guba, 1985), in which the researcher seeks verification by going back to study participants, can be an important step in guarding against researcher bias. It also represents a logical extension of the close relationship between the researcher and the respondent. However, it also raises a number of questions, making it one of the more problematic rigor strategies both in theory and practice.

Member checks shift authority toward participants, thereby properly challenging the status of researcher as infallible observer. Two problems emerge from this, however. First is the basic issue of what exactly members are checking. If asked to review their own interview transcript or personal case summary, participants' authority is rarely challenged. But member checks often refer to cross-case interpretation; it is reasonable to wonder if an individual respondent can (or should) be expected to pass judgment on findings involving many hours of immersion and synthesis. Second, member checking (as with triangulation) implies that a single "reality" can be captured (albeit this time by participants rather than by peers or others; Sandelowski, 1993). Thus, respondents may disagree with a study's findings not because the findings are inaccurate, but because respondents have their own standpoints and realities, all of which may change over time (Rolfe, 2006).

The practicalities of member checking can be daunting. Some respondents do not want to be bothered or will hastily "rubber stamp" whatever is in front of them. Others may not wish to revisit their earlier statements and emotions. A program director, for example, may have second thoughts about what she has told you about mismanagement by mid-level administrators. For some studies, logistical barriers or gatekeeper issues prevent going back. Data collection in a faraway location, for example, may preclude revisiting participants in person. Member checks also fall into a gray area when it comes to human subjects committee oversight. Can they be considered part of the approved interview protocol and thus not require additional consent? What happens if and when member checking verges into new data collection? This is a fine line that cannot often be predicted or managed in advance.

As with triangulation, it is when member checking produces conflicting perspectives that problems arise. This can prompt revisiting the data and generating new interpretations, but the researcher may wish to stick to his viewpoint (and explain why he feels this way). Novice qualitative researchers should take heart: Non-negotiable disagreements during member checking are rare. In any event, the act of consulting with respondents—regardless of the outcome—affirms their dignity as research partners.

Negative Case Analysis

Although discussed in Chapter 8, the importance of negative case analysis bears repeating here as a strategy for rigor (see Figure 9.1). Just as the PDS group challenges a researcher to explore personal biases, negative case analysis puts the onus on the researcher to operate in a critically self-reflective way when analyzing and interpreting the data. As such, it enhances fairness (i.e., giving equitable attention to differing viewpoints and avoiding favoritism and lopsided interpretations; Morrow, 2005).

Auditing—Leaving a Decision Trail

Leaving an audit or decision trail means adopting a spirit of openness and documenting each step taken in data collection and analysis (Lincoln & Guba, 1985). The components of an audit trail include raw data as well as memos noting decisions made during data collection, coding, and analysis. Although it is not intended for exact replication, an audit trail does enhance *reproducibility*; that is, another researcher is able to use it to verify the findings (Schwandt & Halpern, 1988).

In a sense, auditing is a meta-strategy for enhancing rigor because it documents that the other strategies—prolonged engagement, peer support, member checks, triangulation, and negative case analysis—have been used appropriately. Box 9.1 provides an exemplary article in which the authors (Morrow & Smith, 1995) successfully applied (and wrote about) all six strategies for rigor.

Box 9.1 Strategies for Rigor in Action: An Exemplar Study

A sure sign of the maturity of qualitative methods is the growing number of rigorous and transparent studies in the published literature. One of these, a study of women who survived childhood sexual abuse, offers particularly thorough description. Conducted by Susan Morrow and Mary Lee Smith (1995), the study is one of few that have used—and reported on—all six strategies for rigor. Here is what they tell the reader:

Prolonged Engagement—The authors report multiple interviews and more than 16 months of varied encounters with participants.

Peer Debriefing—Morrow met weekly with an interdisciplinary qualitative research collective where members shared feedback on their data collection and analysis procedures.

Triangulation—The authors used multiple sources of data, including in-depth interviews with 11 survivors; videotapes of a 10-week focus group consisting of a subset of 7 interviewees; documents such as participants' journals; and field notes and a self-reflective journal kept by Morrow.

Member Checking—At the conclusion of the focus group, all seven members were invited to become participant coresearchers; of these, four accepted and received a brief introduction to grounded theory analysis. Over the course of a year, they worked with the authors on member checking, analyzing videotapes of their respective group sessions, and developing codes and categories.

Negative Case Analysis—Acknowledging a "human cognitive bias toward confirmation" (Morrow & Smith, 1995, p. 26), the authors report that they actively searched for disconfirming evidence, including consulting with participants on discrepant findings.

Auditing—The authors kept detailed analytic and self-reflective memos to document their progress. Large poster boards with movable tags were used to arrange and rearrange codes and categories. The audit trail consisted of chronological narratives of their activities as well as a complete list of the 166 codes that formed the basis of the analyses.

In addition, Morrow and Smith (1995) address *evidentiary adequacy* by reporting on the breadth of the data: 220 hours of audio- and videotaping, 165 hours of interviews, 24 hours of group sessions, and 25 hours of follow-up interactions over a period of 16 months. Data for analysis exceeded 2,000 pages of transcriptions, field notes, and documents.

Questions of Rigor in Community-Based Participatory Research

Given the central premise of community-based participatory research (CBPR)—sharing control with community members—one may reasonably fear a potential loss of methodological rigor (Allison & Rootman, 1996). Community partners are not likely to have knowledge of research methods or the inclination to accept all of the demands incurred by research protocols. Moreover, the fact that CBPR prioritizes community empowerment can conflict with the researcher's orientation to drawing conclusions that are empirically based, regardless of whether they conform to advocacy goals.

This tension between rigor and relevance, found in all research, is front and center in CBPR. While the researcher's career advancement depends on adherence to standards of scientific peer review, community members understandably may not share this point of view. Too often viewed as a zero-sum game—more community involvement equals less scientific rigor—CBPR is more appropriately viewed as a balancing act than an "either-or" proposition. Although ultimate resolution of the rigor-versus-relevance balancing act depends on the particular circumstances of a study, a few recommendations can be made. First, rigor in CBPR takes dedication, time, and patience. Community members have a right to know and question the study's methods, and when possible, to actively participate in their development and implementation. If community members seek to veto some aspect of the proposed study, the researcher must find a way to either dissuade them respectfully or accede to their wishes and try another route. Second, the most demanding and distancing research designs are a difficult fit with CBPR, especially in the early stages when community buy-in is critical. Thus, an experimental trial to test an innovative program is far more likely to be successful if implemented after a period of community involvement and collaboration. (This is yet another reason for using qualitative methods in CBPR, especially in the early stages.) Finally, threats to the rigor of a CBPR study are greatest when time is short and results are needed quickly. Successful CBPR projects are built upon long-term commitments and mutual learning; i.e., researchers learn about the community, its needs and priorities, and community partners learn about research methods and how they can be harnessed to meet those needs.

Strategies for Rigor in Differing Qualitative Approaches

Some types of rigor strategies are a better fit than others, depending on the type of qualitative approach being used. As alluded to in the above section, CBPR is a natural fit with member checking, but other strategies are plausible, too. Ethnographic research depends first and foremost on prolonged engagement, but it does not preclude using the other strategies. Case study and grounded theory analyses can also benefit from using any of the six strategies, with data triangulation leading the way in case studies and negative case analysis historically allied with grounded theory. A reliance upon texts among narrative approaches makes data triangulation unlikely and negative case analysis inappropriate (since such approaches are not intended to produce explanation), but member checking is plausible. In phenomenological approaches, peer debriefing and auditing are considered potentially contaminating influences that interfere with the search for deep structures of meaning.

Guidelines for Appraising the Quality of a Study: Adequacy Is Key

Appraising the quality of a study goes beyond documenting which strategies for rigor will be (or were) pursued and how. As shown in Box 9.2, skeptical reviewers, whether one's colleagues or "outside" experts, often pose questions that the qualitative researcher would be wise to anticipate. Over the years, a number of checklists for quality have emerged to guide discerning readers (Inui & Frankel, 1991; Patton, 2002; Sandelowski & Barroso, 2002). Cutting across these guidelines are a few central concerns: Are the findings grounded in the data? How were the inevitable intrusions of bias addressed? Were decisions about sampling and analysis reasonable and logical? How systematic and auditable were the study's procedures? Are the interpretations strong and insightful?

Erickson (1986) summed it up as *adequacy*—of data richness, data variety, disconfirming evidence, and interpretations. Existing as a kind of transcendent criteria, adequacy is not about quantity but, rather, sufficiency. Its achievement is rarely predictable in advance but is enhanced considerably by taking the actions described in this chapter.

Box 9.2 Addressing Questions From Skeptical Reviewers

Experienced qualitative researchers are accustomed to answering questions from colleagues, many well-meaning but nonetheless persistent in their skepticism. The following are some common queries. The more you can anticipate these, the better prepared you will be to explain not only your study but also all qualitative studies.

- "How can this study be generalizable with that sample size?"
- "Where are your hypotheses?"
- "Why isn't this more objective?"
- "Will sample attrition be a problem with so few in the study?"
- "Why can't you be more forthcoming about what your findings will look like in advance?"
- "How is this different from journalism?"

The "before and after" distinction is important here. Although qualitative researchers might include strategies for rigor in their description of methods before the study begins, equally if not more important is the documentation of what actually transpired in the study. Box 9.3 features brief descriptions of studies in which the authors did just this.

Box 9.3 Some Examples of Methodological Transparency

Space limitations and confusion over what to include or exclude often lead researchers to shortchange their methods descriptions. Some have published journal articles devoted to explicating their methods so that others can learn from their experiences. The following are a few concrete examples of transparency in methods descriptions.

- Cashman and colleagues (2008) give brief reports of four CBPR projects and describe how they met the challenges of jointly analyzing data and disseminating outcomes. The location and focus of the projects included

(Continued)

(Continued)

the following: New Mexico (tribal public health infrastructure), Detroit (social determinants of health), North Carolina (Latino men and HIV risk), and New York City (environmental health). Each had different methods, and each found ways to benefit from complementary skills of community members and researchers.

- Chiovitti and Piran (2003) used their grounded theory study of psychiatric ward nurses to illustrate the step-by-step process of generating a theory, checking it with study participants, and establishing auditability and transferability.
- Correll (1995) carried out an ethnographic study of an online "lesbian cafe" and candidly discussed the challenges of doing research in cyberspace, including what "observation" means, the ethical challenges of maintaining anonymity in an open-access site, and the creative use of emoticons and other text notes that are unfamiliar in traditional data analyses.
- Bowen (2006) wrote of the challenges of using grounded theory in an antipoverty project in Jamaica. Following a constructivist paradigm, he applied sensitizing concepts such as empowerment and social capital while developing a grounded theory of stakeholder collaboration in development work. Bowen used hindsight to reflect on his study and the ways in which a priori concepts (prior knowledge) blended with emergent findings.

Summary and Concluding Thoughts

This chapter has revolved around a few main points: (1) Methodological rigor and evaluative standards are needed in qualitative research; (2) evidence of quality emerging from a completed study is not the same as building into a study's design deliberate efforts to improve quality; (3) achieving rigor can be enhanced by using one or more of six strategies developed explicitly for qualitative studies; and (4) a study's trustworthiness depends on fairness and ethical conduct as well as rigor. Peer reviews serve the primary gatekeeping function in determining rigor and trustworthiness. By implication, such reviews are dependent on a set of criteria that serve as guideposts rather than stringent prescriptions. That there is little consensus on what these criteria should be constitutes an ongoing conundrum for qualitative researchers.

By now, the reader may be wondering if any stone has been left unturned in the search for rigor. On the plus side, this pursuit is a decidedly "low tech" enterprise, requiring neither technical savvy nor fancy software (nor footwork). On the challenging side, there can be difficulties along the way. Setting up peer debriefing groups can tax the resources of a researcher, school, or department. The time commitment necessary for prolonged engagement requires shifting one's life around to support absences from work and home. Miles and Huberman (1994) estimate a 20% increase in time expenditures imposed by documentation for an audit trail. Finally, member checking and triangulation can bring out discrepancies and interpretive conflicts that are not easily resolved.

Despite these complicating factors and demands, rigor is essential to all forms of empirical research, whether quantitative or qualitative. However the evaluative standards are defined and applied, it is difficult to justify a non-rigorous study as having relevance.

EXERCISES

1. This can be done alone or in a group. Select and read a qualitative study from one of the following journals: *Qualitative Health Research, Social Science & Medicine,* or the *American Journal of Public Health.* Note what (if any) strategies for rigor the authors mention in discussing their methods and findings.

2. Read the article titled "Reading Qualitative Studies" by Sandelowski and Barroso (available online in the *International Journal of Qualitative Methods, 1*(1), 2002, at www.ualberta.ca/~iiqm/backissues/1_1Final/1_1toc.html). Following their guidelines, choose a published study and critique it. What are some of the topics most often neglected by authors?

3. Develop an idea for a study you would like to conduct in the future. Which strategies for rigor would be most appropriate?

4. In a group, discuss the three threats to trustworthiness (reactivity, researcher bias, and respondent bias) and how they differ in quantitative versus qualitative studies. Are quantitative studies more vulnerable to some threats than others? What about qualitative studies?

Additional Readings

Altheide, D. L., & Johnson, J. M. (1994). Criteria for assessing interpretive validity in qualitative research. In N. K. Denzin & Y. S. Lincoln (Eds.), *Handbook of qualitative research* (pp. 485–499). Thousand Oaks, CA: Sage.

Davies, D., & Dodd, J. (2002). Qualitative research and the question of rigor. *Qualitative Health Research, 12*(2), 279–289.

Devers. K. (1999). How will we know "good" qualitative research when we see it? Beginning the dialogue in health services research. *Health Services Research, 34,* 1153–1187.

Kidd, P. S., & Parshall, M. B. (2000). Getting the focus and the group: Enhancing analytical rigor in focus group research. *Qualitative Health Research, 10*(3), 293–308.

LeCompte, M. D., & Goetz, J. P. (1984). Problems of reliability and validity in ethnographic research. *Review of Educational Research, 52,* 31–60.

Leininger, M. (1994). Evaluation criteria and critique of qualitative research studies. In J. M. Morse (Ed.), *Critical issues in qualitative research methods* (pp. 95–115). Thousand Oaks, CA: Sage.

Lincoln, Y. S. (1995). Emerging criteria for quality in qualitative and interpretative research. *Qualitative Inquiry, 1*(3), 275–289.

Marshall, C. (1990). Goodness criteria: Are they objective or judgment calls? In E. G. Guba (Ed.), *The paradigm dialog* (pp. 188–197). Newbury Park, CA: Sage.

Maxwell, J. A. (1992). Understanding and validity in qualitative research. *Harvard Educational Review, 62*(3), 279–300.

Morrow, S. L. (2005). Quality and trustworthiness in qualitative research in counseling psychology. *Journal of Counseling Psychology, 52,* 250–260.

Morse, J. M., Barrett, M., Mayan, M., Olsen, K., & Spiers, S. (2002). Verification strategies for establishing reliability and validity in qualitative research. *International Journal of Qualitative Methods, 1,* Article 2.

Sandelowski, M. (1993). Rigor, or rigor mortis: The problem of rigor in qualitative research revisited. *Advances in Nursing Science, 6,* 1–8.

Sandelowski, M., & Barroso, J. (2002). Reading qualitative studies. *International Journal of Qualitative Methods, 1*(1), Article 5.

Seale, C. (1999). *The quality of qualitative research.* London: Sage.

Seale C. (2002). Quality issues in qualitative inquiry. *Qualitative Social Work, 1*(1), 97–110.

Whittemore, R., Chase, S. K., & Mandle, C. (2001). Validity in qualitative research. *Qualitative Health Research, 11*(4), 522–527.

10

Telling the Story

Writing Up the Qualitative Study

Qualitative researchers who have a talent for writing are fortunate souls. For most, however, writing up a qualitative study takes a good deal of effort—it is a craft to be learned and honed over time.

If the act of writing up quantitative research is pro forma and somewhat anticlimactic (a well-conducted study can usually survive a poor write-up), it is the climactic event in qualitative research (Padgett, 2004c). Studies are "vast conversations with dispersed others" (Flaherty, 2002, p. 510), and qualitative researchers have an obligation to ensure the conversation is lively and thought-provoking.

The ideal scenario in writing up a qualitative study involves maintaining a clear alignment between one's choice of method and the explicit terminology used to describe the study and its procedures. (If invoked, epistemology should also be compatible.) Sandelowksi and Barroso (2003) examined a number of qualitative studies and found that this ideal was rarely attained. Instead, authors obscured the diversity of their approaches through generic description, many relying on what appeared to be variations of content analysis. For studies that offered specifics, there was frequently a disconnect between self-labeling and reality—for example, a study that was ostensibly phenomenological used a version of grounded theory.

Two rather obvious suggestions can help prepare for writing. First, read as many good qualitative studies as possible. Exemplary articles have been cited throughout this book, and several suggestions for full-length monographs are listed at the end of this chapter. Reading and absorbing both the form and substance of qualitative studies will expose you to the many options available for the study write-up and help you to develop your own style. Second, begin writing early and build in plenty of time for editing and polishing. It is better to write even when one does not feel like it than to wait for a lightning bolt of inspiration to strike (Wolcott, 2009). Start with an outline and flesh it out as you go. Difficulties in writing are less often due to "writer's block" than to "idea block" (Lofland & Lofland, 1995, p. 205). The self-selection process leading individuals toward qualitative research tends to favor creative, abstract thinkers. The challenge is to keep those ideas and abstractions firmly grounded in the data.

Deciding on an Approach

Many qualitative researchers have shared their own strategies for writing, including Richardson (2005), van Manen (2006), Weiss (1994), and Wolcott (2009). In reviewing their works and through my own experience, I have identified four decisions facing the qualitative researcher approaching the write-up phase. The first two of these—deciding on the audience for the study and how (if at all) to describe the researcher's role in the report—are common to all write-ups even if not made explicit. The other two decisions—whether and how to use numbers and how to address coauthorship—may or may not be encountered depending upon the nature of the study.

Targeting the Audience

Qualitative reports have the potential to reach broad audiences with their accessible, almost literary style of presentation. Some of the best qualitative studies began as research reports but crossed over to gain wide and lasting public appeal. Several of the monographs listed at the end of this chapter have had such an impact. Qualitative studies may be written up for a number of purposes and audiences. For academic audiences—doctoral dissertation committees, journal editors, and conference attendees—the write-up is pitched at a high level to ensure that new knowledge is evident. Evaluative reports are usually written in more pragmatic language (less academic-speak) and are structured to provide concrete suggestions for improving policies and practices. When a study is commissioned and funded, the sponsoring organization usually wants the researcher to assess specific problems and recommend solutions. As a target audience, the sponsor may also try to influence how the study is written. It is always a good idea to consult with key stakeholders, but the researcher must assume ultimate responsibility for producing a report that is as balanced and accurate as possible.

Box 10.1   Beyond Scientific Publication: Reaching New Audiences in Public Health Research

Like their colleagues in other health professions, public health researchers adhere to a scientific agenda dependent on peer-reviewed journal publications. Recent years, however, have brought greater attention to the democratization of information including dissemination in a variety of formats for diverse audiences. The Community Alliance for Research and Engagement (CARE) at Yale University has produced an excellent online resource for disseminating findings through print media, television, radio, the Internet, or a community forum. Reports may take the form of press releases, brochures, flyers, policy briefs, newsletters, web postings, and podcasts. The document, which can be found at www.researchtoolkit.org/primer/docs/CARE%20 Research%20Dissemination%20Guide.pdf, offers numerous examples ranging from executive summaries to thank you letters sent to participants. The increasing sophistication of public health's image, no doubt assisted by media attention to large-scale philanthropic endeavors targeting AIDS, malaria, and other diseases, has made multimedia dissemination de rigueur.

The Researcher's Role in the Report

The de facto stance for a qualitative researcher up to the 1970s was largely that of an omniscient but invisible outsider. Characterized as "Realist Tales" by Van Maanen (1988), these earlier studies took scant notice of the researcher's role—to use first-person pronouns was an unthinkable breach of etiquette. Authors of Realist Tales spent many private hours regaling colleagues and students with stories of their experiences in the field but then edited such stories out of their writing as unseemly self-indulgence (Van Maanen, 1988).

The rise of constructivism and postmodernism directly challenged this state of affairs. To postmodern critics, the human emotions stirred by fieldwork were squeezed out of the report by a "Doctrine of Immaculate Perception" (Van Maanen, 1988, p. 73) that obscured vividness and ambiguity. In the meantime, academic and general audiences have come to accept the use of first-person pronouns (at least in qualitative studies). In some quarters, the pendulum has swung all the way to the researcher as the focus of interest with autoethnographies, memoirs, and other "Confessional Tales" (Van Maanen, 1988) taking center stage.

It is abundantly clear that the researcher is a key actor in the qualitative study and should not be hidden or edited out of the final report. What remains open to question is how prominently the researcher's role should be featured. If taken too far, reflexivity produces tedious self-absorption. However, much of one's experience in the field—failures as well as successes—can be pertinent to the credibility of the study.

The decision about how much personal information and experience to include in the final report is influenced not only by one's epistemological stance, but also by the intended audience and the outlet for the report's dissemination. Whereas some audiences might appreciate full reflexivity, practitioners and policy makers are likely to find it self-indulgent and distracting. The form reflexivity takes can range from brief mention of one's stance at the report's outset to a thorough description of how the researcher entered the field, interacted with participants, and grappled with potential intrusions of bias. The latter, often drawn from the personal journal or diary kept during the study, situates the author as an active participant in the study.

Journal articles tend to be less evidently self-reflexive, in part due to the shortage of space and the need to give the methods and findings their full due. Full-length reports (e.g., dissertations and books) may have the researcher's role threaded throughout, or they may place it in a separate section or appendix. A candid and lengthy appendix can be found in Mitch Duneier's book *Sidewalk* (1999), in which he discusses the origin and evolution of his study of homeless men in Greenwich Village, New York. In their write-ups, most qualitative researchers give the lion's share of space to the data and findings without trying to hide their role. Harking back to the previous chapter, including a section on strategies for rigor used during the study is an excellent vehicle for addressing concerns about potential biases.

Using Numbers in the Report

Perhaps less weighty is the decision about whether and how to use numbers in writing the final report. Few qualitative studies give much credence to numbers, but some findings can be amenable to quantifying. As discussed in Chapter 8, a few caveats pertain to using numbers in qualitative studies. First, given nonrepresentative and small sample sizes, numerical findings can give a false impression of precision where none exists. Sometimes, using "most" or "some" is sufficient (Weiss, 1994). Another caveat is this: Many important findings in qualitative studies were not routinely elicited but emerged serendipitously and voluntarily. As such, any count of the number of respondents who gave certain information is probably an undercount and is thus misleading for those who assume it is a "true" measure of frequency. These caveats do not mean that all numerical indicators should be banned from qualitative reports—at a minimum, demographic characteristics usually get reported in frequencies and percentages. They do, however, draw attention to the risks of using numbers.

Coauthorship in Qualitative Studies

Qualitative research has a long tradition of solo work. A trend toward teamwork, however, has made coauthorship a common endeavor. This trend has been especially evident in public health where research collaboration has long been a common by-product of working in multidisciplinary settings promoting health among diverse populations.

Qualitative collaborations are multifaceted and interwoven—almost every phase informing and being informed by every other. This seamless quality carries over into writing the report. In contrast, quantitative studies and reports can usually be broken down into discrete tasks and assigned to team members according to their role on the project and their individual strengths.

Deciding on authorship in any type of study can be tricky. For example, do the most senior members of the team have first dibs on authorship (especially the rank of first author)? Or should authorial rank be strictly a matter of who did what and how much? Research and professional ethics dictate that the first author will have done the most work, including writing the study report. Coauthorship down the line is apportioned according to relative contribution. To deal with the inevitable confusion, many journals publish guidelines and require coauthors to sign off on what they did to earn their place in the hierarchy. Thankfully, the days of a "free ride" (where the lab director or department chair was automatically given coauthor status) are over.

The egalitarian ethos of qualitative inquiry affects the teamwork, making leadership roles less foreordained and subverting attempts to impose decisions based on seniority alone. This is especially evident in participatory approaches where researchers and community partners must negotiate authorship as well as decide who will represent the project in public gatherings, conference presentations, and the like. For the latter, it is not unusual to see two individuals—a researcher and community partner—step forward together. With regard to the former, it is more common to see the researcher as the lead author with community partners listed as coauthors and included in all phases of the write-up. Gaining experience in research methods, writing and public advocacy enhances capacity building in the community and levels the playing field such that the researchers share control over how and when the study is presented to outsiders. A project with community partners and researchers alternating as first author would be the ideal scenario.

Organizing the Report—Key Components

The amount of creative latitude in writing up a qualitative report depends on its purpose and intended audience. Still, most qualitative reports follow the same format as quantitative ones, as described here:

1. *Background and Theoretical Context.* Here, the authors describe the phenomenon of interest, including a rationale for the study and its use of qualitative methods. The literature review that follows places the study within a theoretical and empirical context. The review may separately cover qualitative studies to further situate the study and its potential contribution. Theoretical influences and conceptual frameworks are presented along with the requisite caveat that they are not driving (or confining) the study. This section is a sustained argument undergirding the study. Critiquing the methods and conclusions of empirical work is fair game, but the argument and rationale is more about gaps in knowledge than errors or incompetence in previous research (Silverman, 2006).

This section usually ends with an overarching study question or two and the study's research questions.

2. *Methods*. This section typically begins by introducing the reader to the specific method (grounded theory, ethnography, narrative analysis, etc.) with liberal citations of methodologists' published work in the area. It then gives a detailed description of how the study's goals were accomplished (which often diverges from the original proposal or plan). Here, the author describes the hows, whens, and whys of the study: its site and sample selection, entering the field and establishing rapport, data collection procedures, storing and managing data, data analyses, human subjects and ethical considerations, and strategies used to enhance rigor. The authors should be forthcoming about the qualifications of those involved in data collection and analysis.

3. *Findings*. Qualitative researchers may use a variety of means to report findings, ranging from graphic displays such as charts, matrices, and maps to lists or schemas of codes and themes (usually illustrated by selected quotes from the transcripts). They may also present case vignettes or typologies to illustrate major categories or themes.

4. *Conclusions and Recommendations*. Highlights of the study bear repeating here to remind the reader of the study's goals, to summarize how these goals were achieved, and to discuss the study's limitations. The implications of the findings are also important. How do they advance knowledge? What are their applications to practice and policy? Finally, what are suggested directions for future research?

Here are a few additional pointers: (1) Make clear distinctions among these four sections—for example, do not introduce new findings in the conclusion section; (2) use headings and subheadings to structure the report and to serve as signposts leading the way; (3) cite sources liberally and often—it is far better to over-cite than to risk even the appearance of plagiarism; (4) carefully choose your title (see Box 10.2 for suggested guidelines); and (5) aim for maximum transparency and elucidation. As discussed in Chapter 8, thoroughness in describing one's methods and findings enhances confidence in the study and helps with the larger and still-needed task of demystifying qualitative research. A qualitative study may have many or few limitations, but small sample size and lack of generalizability should not be considered among them. Unless it was also a single-interview study of a few participants (thus shortchanging the study on depth and breadth), one need not apologize for sample size. And, since "generalizability" is not a standard to which qualitative studies must adhere, it makes little sense to consider it an inherent limitation. Still, a prudent researcher might anticipate such objections and provide a brief preemptive explanation with relevant citations.

Box 10.2   Choosing the Right Title

Ideally, the study's title should be catchy but not frivolous. Anthropologists have a long tradition of two-part titles, one phrase seriously descriptive and the other intended for broader appeal. Here is a partial listing of article titles from the NYSS:

- "In Their Own Words: Trauma and Substance Abuse in the Lives of Formerly Homeless Women With Serious Mental Illness"
- "Disappearing Acts: The Social Networks of Homeless Individuals With Co-occurring Disorders"
- "There's No Place Like (a) Home: Ontological Security in the Third Decade of the "Homelessness Crisis" in the United States"
- "Engagement and Retention in Care Among Formerly Homeless Adults With Serious Mental illness: Voices From the Margins"

The phrases such as "in their own words" and "voices from the margins" indicated that the study was qualitative (to readers in the predominantly quantitative journals to which they were submitted for publication). Putting the term *qualitative* in the title or in the study's key words (we chose to do the latter) is important—otherwise it will never be retrievable through database searches for qualitative studies (a problem that many scholars of knowledge dissemination bemoan). We were able to use wordplay, for example, "there's no place like (a) home" and "disappearing acts," to emphasize two critical points being made in the studies. Note the use of irony and sarcasm in putting the phrase "homelessness crisis" in quotation marks after noting its 30-year (and counting) duration in the title. Ending this title with "in the United States" was a nod to the international focus of the journal to which it was submitted (*Social Science & Medicine*, one of my personal favorites). Some authors like to use participant quotes in their titles. Boeri's study titled "'Hell, I'm an Addict, But I Ain't No Junkie': An Ethnographic Analysis of Aging

Heroin Users" (2004) is one example of an in vivo–inspired title (albeit a rather long one). Of course, one does not need a snappy phrase every time. Some journals prefer more subdued titles, and some studies are better suited to catchiness than others.

Qualitative Reports Across the Diverse Approaches

Each of the qualitative approaches may have its own writing conventions that represent variations on the format previously described, but the overwhelming majority of qualitative reports rely on narrative with the option of including tables, figures, photographs, and other illustrative graphics. Grounded theory reports typically follow the architecture of the theory or conceptual framework that emerged from the analyses. Thus, categories or themes are listed along with selected quotes to illustrate them. In some instances, the theoretical schema is diagrammed to visually depict the categories, using arrows to indicate the relationships between them. Charmaz (2006) recommends that grounded theorists do not shy away from ambiguities and uncertainties in the report.

Phenomenological reports tend to be prestructured based on their analytic structure. Colaizzi (1978) suggests including tables of themes and significant statements, a format that Beck (1993) followed in her phenomenological study of postpartum depression. Moustakas (1994) gives a detailed set of guidelines for phenomenological reports, including recommending an autobiographical account at the beginning to bracket the researcher. The *Journal of Phenomenological Psychology* contains many examples of this approach.

Ethnographic studies have a tradition of book-length reports, their length deemed necessary to capture the scope of the inquiry. Although many have an engaging storytelling quality, others tend toward the encyclopedic in their amassing of details derived from long hours of participant observation. Early ethnographies had missing or severely truncated sections on methods, but much has changed over the past 20 years as prominent researchers have stepped forward to offer suggestions (LeCompte & Schensul, 2010; Tedlock, 2000).

Narrative approaches often use the *zoom in/zoom out technique* (Czarniawska, 2004) of spotlighting portions of annotated texts and then interpreting their meaning according to the study's specific method (narrative analysis, conversational analysis, or discourse analysis). Published examples of narrative reports show how the authors alternate interpretation with annotated excerpts (Hyden & Overlien, 2004; Riessman, 1993; Sands, 2004). By way of contrast, grounded theory and phenomenological reports place greater emphasis on interpretive structures and use illustrative excerpts.

Case studies may vary considerably in format depending on their design (single versus multiple case) and aims. Stake (2005) describes the basics of a case study report, including a description of the study's purpose (especially the significance of the case or cases), methods, and setting. Because many case studies are used for evaluative purposes or to critically analyze an issue, their write-ups typically include vignettes, quotes, and graphic displays to illustrate the main points and prevent the reader from getting lost in the minutiae of the case.

Balancing Description and Interpretation

The reader has probably surmised by now that a prime source of variation in qualitative reports is how they balance description versus interpretation. This is not a cut-and-dried decision. In Chapter 6 (see Box 6.1), we examined the continuum running from raw description during observation to higher-order levels of abstraction. Inferences and interpretations are drawn from analyzing what is said and observed, but they also derive their power from considerations of what is *not* said or observed as well as the broader context of what is known and what needs to be known. Thus, the fund of knowledge brought to bear by the analytic team—preferably broad as well as deep—profoundly affects the impact of the findings.

Although "analytic excess" (Lofland, 2002, p. 158) robs the report of the rich detail on which it is based, too little analysis severely reduces its impact. Concerned about the latter, anthropologist Clifford Geertz (1973) introduced the term *thick description* to invigorate ethnographic interpretation. Such interpretation involves abstraction and meaning-making. It is not armchair conjecture or theorizing but instead is rooted in prolonged experience with the phenomenon under study.

Ethnographies often blend description with interpretation in a seamless manner, but most qualitative reports present the interpretive structure of the findings interspersed with excerpts of raw data. Creswell (2007), for example, discusses ratios of 70/30 or 60/40 favoring description.

Lofland (2002) settles on roughly the same balance. Yet it is the quality of the interpretation that defines excellence in qualitative studies. As one public health journal editor put it rather bluntly, "the splat of data in a quotation can illustrate a view, illuminate a problem, but it does not amount to analysis" and runs the risk of being a "superficial sound bite" (Daly, 2009, p. 405). The compartmentalization of description and quotes is made worse when the quotes are placed separately rather than interwoven into the text. Thankfully, this format of reporting has become relatively rare (Daly, 2009).

Multiple Findings and Reports: A Growing Phenomenon in Large-Scale Studies

A qualitative or mixed methods study may generate several manuscripts submitted for peer-reviewed journal publication (not to mention yielding up reports to various stakeholders). To avoid self-plagiarizing, or recycling text beyond what is considered fair use in copyright law, researchers should make sure that separate analyses and associated manuscripts are distinct, with minimal overlap or repetition. That said, a large-scale effort or one that extends over a period of time will almost certainly yield a variety of stand-alone findings.

Quantitative researchers have an easier time parsing their data and findings into separate accounts; they can also compact their findings into dense tables of statistics and thereby save space. For qualitative researchers, the turn away from book-length monographs to journal articles spanning different outlets has introduced new problems for reports traditionally characterized by seamless narrative. Here are a few suggestions on how this might be done:

- The findings may be complemented by a separate methodological article discussing some of the innovative techniques being used (if appropriate).
- A mixed methods study's findings might be broken up into their quantitative and qualitative portions (advisable only if there is no intention or need to integrate them).
- Authors may publish reports from a longitudinal study at appropriate junctures or stopping points along the way.

The "prism is turned," and different aspects of the data are rich enough to sustain multiple analyses and reports. This was a fortunate by-product of the expansive scope of the NYSS in which 39 life histories in Phase 1 were followed by a Phase 2 prospective follow-up of 85 formerly home-less individuals who were interviewed at 0, 6, and 12 months and their case managers were interviewed twice. Published reports—which at this writing number 11 journal articles and 3 book chapters—reflect a team effort as well as the generous sharing by study participants.

Writing Stance and Style

Rhetorical Devices Suited to Qualitative Studies

Successful qualitative reports give readers a new perspective and challenge them to think differently. A favorite approach is to debunk or refute cherished notions such as stereotypes and outdated beliefs. Qualitative researchers are justifiably proud of their record of probing beneath the carefully constructed facade and coming up with findings that challenge the status quo. Eric Klinenberg's *Heat Wave* (2002), for example, reports on Chicago's disastrous summer of 1995 as a slow-motion nightmare of public policy failures resulting in the deaths of 700 of the city's most vulnerable and isolated citizens. Here is another example: Hirsch and colleagues (2002) conducted research among couples in rural Mexican villages and found that HIV risk (presented by husbands returning from work in the United States) was paradoxically related to the adoption of romantic notions of marriage by the couples. Romantic marriages, with strong expectations of monogamy, were more likely to lead husbands to secretly visit prostitutes (thereby incurring a greater risk of contracting HIV) than to enter into more stable extramarital relationships.

Qualitative research is tailor-made for rhetorical devices such as *debunking, irony,* and *demystification.* The mother who confesses to loathing her children as much as she loves them and the "lazy" men on the street corner who are really furloughed construction workers—all are stories that need to be told. By doing so, qualitative researchers expose the incongruities and inequities taken for granted in social life.

Some qualitative researchers embrace subtle (and not so subtle) irony in framing the findings, thereby drawing attention to gaps between what was observed and what is widely assumed or "known" (Lofland & Lofland, 1995). As noted by Fine and Martin (1990), Erving Goffman was a master at using irony and sarcasm in his *Asylums* (1961).

Demystification is about enlightenment and clarification. Describing the intricacies of human behavior demands in-depth probing and a willingness to take risks and be open-minded. Reji Mathew, a former doctoral student of mine, chose to study arranged marriage among her fellow South Asians living in the United States. Her in-depth interviews with immigrant women yielded a nuanced portrait of this tradition that belied some of the harsher stereotypes. Rather, these interviews revealed how "arranged introductions" emerged to meet the needs of these modern young women and their families (Mathew, 2008).

There is one more thing for which qualitative reports are ideally suited—giving voice to study participants. More often than not, these individuals and groups have had few opportunities to express themselves in their own words. One of the easiest arguments to make for conducting the NYSS was to urge that the opinions of the homeless mentally ill were worth listening to—and that such firsthand accounts were largely missing from the voluminous literature on the problems of homelessness and serious mental illness.

Writing Style: Creating Rhythm and Flow

Most successful qualitative reports have a rhythmic quality, weaving excerpts from the data into an exposition of the study's themes and interpretation. Such reports are confident but not pompous, compelling but not argumentative. The length of the raw excerpt depends on the approach taken by the researcher; care should be taken to avoid breaching confidentiality when making this decision. Most qualitative studies juxtapose small chunks of data—verbatim quotes or brief vignettes—with interpretation. Narrative analyses use lengthier excerpts so that the arc of the story can be presented from beginning to end (Riessman, 1993). Excerpts should push the narrative forward, not be a diversion. McCracken (1988) likened this process to a small plane practicing takeoffs and landings. The plane gains altitude (interpretation and exposition of study themes), but it also repeatedly touches down on the landing strip (excerpting of raw data). The researcher aspires to flawless takeoffs and landings.

Use of Metaphors and Other Tropes

One of the more enjoyable aspects of writing (and reading) qualitative reports is the use of *metaphors*. As examples, Erving Goffman (1961) described the "careers" of mental patients, Sandelowski and Jones (1995) told of the "healing fictions" that pregnant women devise to explain a diagnosis of fetal anomalies, and Liebow (1993) portrayed the "little murders of everyday life" endured by homeless African American women. Respondents may themselves use metaphors, whether commonplace ("walking on thin ice") or highly imaginative (the gardening metaphor invoked by African American women with breast cancer described in Chapter 8). Other tropes used to spice up a qualitative narrative include *turning points* and *epiphanies* (Denzin, 1989), each calling to mind those critical moments when events converge to alter a person's life. Such figures of speech give a transcendent quality to the study and its interpretations.

The Ultimate Goal—Dissemination of the Study Findings

Dissemination has to be the ultimate goal of all studies. Researchers have a number of reasons (excuses?) for not disseminating. Some apply unrealistic standards to their own work and become paralyzed by them. There is also the fear of failure. As Robert Weiss (1994) noted, "writing is exposure" (p. 205), and few exposures are more humbling than submitting manuscripts and reports for review. However, to shelve the data and findings betrays the trust of the study's participants who had generously shared their stories and lives in the first place. CBPR in particular subscribes to a value of wide and accessible dissemination (Chen, Diaz, Lucas, & Rosenthal, 2010).

As discussed earlier in Box 10.1, modes of dissemination can vary tremendously. Qualitative reports are especially suited for publication in book form because of their length—the "classic" works in ethnography were all books. Writing for peer-reviewed journal publication, accorded the highest prestige in academic fields outside of the humanities, is the most challenging form of dissemination. For some qualitative researchers, squeezing findings into 25 or fewer pages compromises the study's integrity. For most, however, the prestige and career enhancement make it worth the effort. Although the situation has improved significantly in recent years, the fact that many reviewers and journal editors are predominantly quantitative or have difficulty accepting the norms of qualitative scholarship presents barriers to publication. Even qualitative-friendly journals and reviewers must grapple with the lack of consensus on standards for quality and rigor.

On a more upbeat note, professional journals are open to qualitative studies as never before. The listing of journals at the end of Chapter 1 is evidence of this. To their credit, many offer longer word limits for qualitative and mixed methods reports (Daly, 2009). Would-be authors are well advised to scrutinize a journal closely to get a sense of what successful entries look like. The overriding message here is one of tenacity and hope. I like to think that every worthwhile study has a place somewhere in the universe of dissemination options. Journals nowadays have impact scores and rejection rates available to would-be submitters so that they can compile a list of potential outlets based on degree of difficulty as well as fit. If I feel I have an "A list" manuscript, I go for it (and let the reviewers decide). If they do not approve, I go to Plan B or Plan C as the occasion demands. At other times, I may have a more modest effort and will start out with a B- or C-list journal.

Unless explicitly told not to resubmit, I consider rejection letters accompanied by reviewers' comments as open invitations to try again. (I learned this lesson from a more experienced colleague who congratulated me when I dejectedly showed him my first rejection letter.) Most often, the verdict is "revise and resubmit" with no guarantee of publication. Assuming the suggested revisions are reasonable, we faithfully make them and resubmit. If a suggestion appears unreasonable, we politely counterargue that it does not work for the study and hope that the reviewers understand. Morse (2007b) offers some helpful hints from her long-time position as editor of *Qualitative Health Research,* including making sure that the introduction and discussion sections are not lengthy when compared to the results (which should be the longest section of a manuscript). She also urges authors to include interpretation along with quotations and ensure that confidentiality is maintained (e.g., demographic characteristics are presented only in the aggregate). Last but far from least, strong manuscripts must make new and compelling contributions to the literature that are stated explicitly and without reservation. Hubris should not be overbearing, but writing the report is "no time to be humble" (Morse, 2007b, p. 1164) when stating one's claims.

Even when a manuscript is rejected, peer reviewers' comments offer helpful tips for revising and resubmitting it elsewhere. This is especially important advice for researchers early in their careers, since such reviews are a gratis (albeit humbling) way to get advice from experts. Regrettably, qualitative researchers must contend with the same problems afflicting journal publication in general, including slow turnaround times (in which manuscripts are essentially held hostage for months at a time) and the uneven quality of reviews.

One bright note on the horizon is the growth in online and open access venues for dissemination. Online publishing can shorten review and publication delays and expand word limits without incurring additional costs. Noteworthy examples include *The Qualitative Report, Forum: Qualitative Social Research (Forum: Qualitative Sozialforschung)*, and the *International Journal of Qualitative Methods*. Electronic access will undoubtedly grow in the future, although the challenges of providing rigorous peer reviews will remain.

Summary and Concluding Thoughts

This chapter has offered a number of suggestions for writing the qualitative report, all proffered in the spirit of "take what is useful and applicable for your needs." Much depends on the structure, format, and style of the writing. At the same time, writing for show rather than substance belies a lack of seriousness and purpose.

The decisions start early and pivot around questions of audience, researcher reflexivity, use of numbers, and divvying up authorship responsibilities. Most write-ups follow the conventional outline (introduction, methods, findings, and conclusions) but can vary depending on which qualitative approach is used and how much space is available for the report.

Stylistically, a qualitative report is an extended argument that also tells a story. In a rhythmic fashion, it blends description and interpretation. To enliven the argument and make it more compelling, qualitative writers use a number of rhetorical devices including metaphors, irony, and other tropes. With the exception of method-specific terminology such as "constant comparative analysis" or "bracketing," the writing should have minimal jargon and be understandable to a broad audience. Intense scholarly works such as dissertations have to employ a higher level of discourse, but they need not be obscurantist. Successful qualitative studies are rigorous, but they are also a good read, spirited and thought-provoking. The researcher's capacity to be surprised and to present serendipitous findings in an engaging manner can make the difference between a ho-hum report and one that grabs an audience and stays with them.

Finally, it is imperative that researchers disseminate their work. Every well-conducted qualitative study has a home out there, whether it is in a top-tier journal or one farther down the prestige hierarchy. As the field of public health goes global, research dissemination in a variety of formats, languages, and mediums is a must. Without dissemination, all of the hard work that came before and all of the cumulative growth of knowledge that can come after are imperiled.

EXERCISES

1. Go to the website of a public health journal and locate a qualitative or mixed methods study using key word search techniques. Bring the article to class. In class discussion, highlight the style of writing used in the article. Do the authors use metaphors or other narrative techniques to get their point across? Do they use numbers, tables, or figures? If so, how?

2. Locate the journal's guidelines for authors submitting manuscripts. Do they include adequate description regarding what the journal expects? Do they include guidelines for assigning rank of coauthorship? Is information provided on the journal's rejection rate or other aspects of its impact?

3. Go to the following web page: www.researchtoolkit.org/primer/docs/CARE %20Research%20Dissemination%20Guide.pdf (mentioned in Box 10.1) and follow the guidelines for writing a press release for local media describing the findings from the article you selected.

4. From the list of monographs at the end of this chapter, check one out from the library and answer the following questions: Is there a chapter or appendix on methods? Does the author talk about his or her role in the study? If so, how much detail is offered? Are figures, tables, and/or photographs used? If so, how do these visual displays help tell the story?

Additional Readings

Janesick, V. J. (2004). *"Stretching" exercises for qualitative researchers* (2nd ed.). Thousand Oaks, CA: Sage.

Padgett, D. K. (2004). Spreading the word: Writing and disseminating qualitative studies. In D. K. Padgett (Ed.), *The qualitative research experience* (pp. 285–296). Belmont, CA: Thomson.

Prendergast, C. (2004). The typical outline of an ethnographic research publication. *Teaching Sociology, 32*(3), 322–327.

Richardson, L. (2005). Writing: A method of inquiry. In N. K. Denzin & Y. S. Lincoln (Eds.), *The SAGE handbook of qualitative research* (3rd ed., pp. 959–978). Thousand Oaks, CA: Sage.

Van Manen, M. (2006). Writing qualitatively, or the demands of writing. *Qualitative Health Research, 16,* 713–722.

Wolcott, H. F. (2009). *Writing up qualitative research* (3rd ed.). Thousand Oaks, CA: Sage.

Selected Monographs

Early Classics

Becker, H., Geer, B., Hughes, E., & Strauss, A. (1961). *Boys in white: Student culture in medical school.* Chicago: University of Chicago Press.

Bosk, C. L. (1979). *Forgive and remember: Managing medical failure.* Chicago: University of Chicago Press.

Estroff, S. (1981). *Making it crazy.* Berkeley: University of California Press.

Gans, H. (1962). *The urban villagers: Group and class in the life of Italian-Americans.* New York: The Free Press.

Goffman, E. (1961). *Asylums: Essays on the social situation of mental patients and other inmates.* Garden City, NY: Basic Books.

Humphries, L. (1970). *Tearoom trade: Impersonal sex in public places.* Chicago: Aldine.

Liebow, E. (1967). *Talley's corner: A study of Negro street corner men.* Boston: Little, Brown.

Lynd, R. S., & Lynd, H. M. (1956). *Middletown: A study in modern American culture.* New York: Harcourt Brace.

Myerhoff, B. (1978). *Number our days: A triumph of continuity and culture among Jewish old people in an urban ghetto.* New York: Simon & Schuster.

Nash, J. C. (1979). *We eat the mines and the mines eat us: Dependency and exploitation in Bolivian tin mines.* New York: Columbia University Press.

Painter, N. I. (1979). *The narrative of Hosea Hudson: His life as a Negro communist in the south.* Cambridge, MA: Harvard University Press.

Powdermaker, H. (1966). *Stranger and friend: The way of an anthropologist.* New York: Norton.

Scheper-Hughes, N. (1981). *Saints, scholars, and schizophrenics: Mental illness in rural Ireland.* Berkeley: University of California Press.

Stack, C. (1974). *All our kin. Strategies for survival in a black community.* New York: Harper Colophon.

Whyte, W. F. (1955). *Street corner society* (2nd ed.). Chicago: University of Chicago Press.

Later Examples

Anderson, E. (1999). *Code of the street: Decency, violence, and the moral life of the inner city.* New York: Norton.

Bourgois, P. (1995). *In search of respect: Selling crack in El Barrio.* New York: Cambridge University Press.

Chan, S. (Ed.). (1994). *Hmong means free: Life in Laos and America.* Philadelphia: Temple University Press.

Duneier, M. (1999). *Sidewalk.* New York: Farrar, Straus & Giroux.

Gourdine, A. K. (2002). *The difference place makes: Gender, sexuality, and diaspora identity.* Columbus: Ohio State University Press.

Hall, T. (2001). *Better times than this: Youth homelessness in Britain.* London: Pluto Press.

Hays, S. (2003). *Flat broke: Women in the age of welfare reform.* New York: Oxford University Press.

Hirsch, J. S. (Ed.). (2009). *The secret: Love, marriage, and HIV.* Nashville, TN: Vanderbilt University Press.

Hochschild, A., with Machung, A. (1989). *The second shift: Inside the two-job marriage.* New York: Avon.

Iversen, R., & Armstrong, A. L. (2006). *Jobs aren't enough: Toward a new economic mobility for low-income families.* Philadelphia: Temple University Press.

Karp, D. A. (1996). *Speaking of sadness: Depression, disconnection, and the meaning of illness.* New York: Oxford University Press.

Klinenberg, E. (2002). *Heat wave: A social autopsy of disaster in Chicago.* Chicago: University of Chicago Press.

Liebow, E. (1993). *Tell them who I am: The lives of homeless women.* New York: Penguin.

Luhrman, T. M. (2000). *Of two minds: The growing disorder in American psychiatry.* New York: Random House.

Martin, E. (2007). *Bipolar expeditions: Mania and depression in America.* Princeton, NJ: Princeton University Press.

Moller, W. D. (2004). *Dancing with broken bones: Portraits of death and dying among inner-city poor.* New York: Oxford University Press.

Newman, K., Fox, C., Roth, W., & Mehta, J. (2005). *Rampage: The social roots of school shootings.* New York: Basic Books.

Oktay, J. (2005). *Breast cancer: Daughters tell their stories.* Binghamton, NY: Haworth Press.

Rhodes, L. (2004). *Total confinement: Madness and reason in the maximum security prison.* Berkeley: University of California Press.

Scheper-Hughes, N. (1992). *Death without weeping: The violence of everyday life in Brazil.* Berkeley: University of California Press.

Venkatesh, S. A. (2006). *Off the books: The underground economy of the urban poor.* Cambridge, MA: Harvard University Press.

Young, A. A. (2004). *The minds of marginalized black men.* Princeton, NJ: Princeton University Press.

Appendix

Writing a Qualitative Methods Proposal for External Funding

With their flexible and rather unpredictable nature, qualitative methods present special challenges when put into proposal form (Morse, 1994). The bar is raised the highest when it comes to external funding, where intense competition combines with a review process steeped in (and thus more favorable to) quantitative methods (Ungar, 2006). And yet qualitative research has attracted external funding for some time and will continue to do so. The trick is to know how to anticipate concerns and optimize the chances of success.

Because this entire book has been dedicated to conducting the type of rigorous qualitative research that can meet the standards of external funders, I will focus in this appendix on the particulars of proposal writing and submission. This discussion is largely based on my experience in collaboratively obtaining grants from the National Cancer Institute, the Centers for Disease Control and Prevention (CDC), and most recently the National Institute of Mental Health (NIMH). I also draw on my experience in reviewing proposals and the experiences of successful colleagues known to me.

I acknowledge at the outset a bias toward National Institutes of Health (NIH) funding because this is where most of my experience lies. Foundations and other nongovernmental sources are equally valuable supporters of high-quality research. Outside of the United States, other nations have a similar mix of governmental and private support for research with varying degrees of openness to qualitative and mixed methods. Success in obtaining external funding for a qualitative study is a challenge, depending in large part on having the right combination of expertise and a strong team of collaborators or consultants. It also involves more than "mere" hard work and dedication—professional contacts, timing, and personal passions also play a role.

There is good news to start out with. First, more funders than ever before are welcoming qualitative and mixed methods proposals. Their reviews may be strenuous and success may be hard to come by, but at least the door is open wider nowadays. Second, qualitative studies can be low-cost enterprises. (A researcher armed with an audio recorder, a laptop computer, and plenty of time is all that is needed.) Smaller grants can go a long way.

Third, assistance is increasingly available to researchers through their own institutions, from funding organizations and via conference workshops. The availability of a mentor can be invaluable. An experienced researcher who has successfully obtained qualitative and mixed methods grants can offer tips on how to frame the issues, how to rationalize the use of qualitative or mixed methods, and how to make the methods section as rigorous as possible. Finally, researchers' home institutions can offer infrastructure supports such as workload reductions, small grants for training or pilot studies, and staff assistance in preparing grant proposals.

External funding offers the "luxury" of having more resources such as personnel, participant incentives, the latest software, and transcription services. It usually brings indirect costs (or overhead) and prestige to one's institution and career advancement for the investigator. The ability to succeed in the highly competitive arena of external funding has become a common expectation of faculty, graduate students, evaluators, and program administrators. One can assume that a proposal will receive close (near-brutal) scrutiny, so thorough preparation begins months in advance.

Writing a qualitative research proposal is an extended effort in persuasion and confidence building in the researcher as well as the methods. Poorly written and poorly argued proposals will not survive the review no matter how worthy the ideas and methods or how seasoned the investigators. I have participated in grant application reviews in which reviewers threw up their hands in frustration over proposals riddled with inconsistencies and errors.

Finding the Right Fit With Funding Priorities: Emerging Opportunities

All of the points made in Chapter 1 apply here regarding reasons for doing qualitative research and the need to choose methods based on one's topic (not the other way around). Here, there is an additional layer of consideration: the potential funder's interests. Foundations tend to be up front about their current priorities, and a check of their website can usually provide this information. A very helpful clearinghouse on foundation support is the Foundation Center at http://foundationcenter.org.

The choice of topic for the proposal may come from personal experience, intellectual curiosity, a passion to change the world, or all of these. What matters most is the ability to shape the topic in such a way that it will attract attention and gain support. Making the case is easier when the study fits with funding priorities. The following discussion is admittedly limited to resources originating primarily in the United States (although many of these are open to non-U.S. researchers and to research topics not confined to the United States). A very helpful online resource that includes sources of public health research funding as well as grant writing tips can be found at http://phpartners.org/grants.html.

The rise of large philanthropic enterprises such as the Bill and Melinda Gates Foundation and the Clinton Foundation has transformed public health research. With an endowment in excess of $34 billion, the Gates Foundation is one of the most sought-after and respected funders of public health research, albeit one that is heavily limited to infectious diseases and biotechnology innovation. In contrast, the Robert Wood Johnson Foundation emphasizes training in the health professions as well as research on childhood obesity and other public health initiatives (http://www.rwjf.org/).

The U.S. National Institutes of Health is one of the largest funders of health research in the world. Although favoring the traditional biomedical model, NIH has funded many qualitative and mixed methods proposals and in 1999 put out a brief guide to assist submitters (http://obssr.od.nih.gov/pdf/Qualitative.PDF). NIH-funded research can range from DNA sequencing to an ethnography of IV drug users. With 27 institutes and centers and a budget exceeding $31 billion annually, the NIH awards 80% of its funds via 50,000 competitive grants to researchers at over 3,000 universities, medical schools, and other research institutions in every U.S. state and around the world (see www.nih.gov for further information).

In recent years, applicants have been required to make a convincing argument about the *public health significance* of their proposed study; it is no longer acceptable to request funds for basic science low-impact studies. In contrast, the federal entity known as SAMHSA (Substance Abuse and Mental Health Services Administration) and its constituent units such as CMHS (Center for Mental Health Services) and CSAT (Center for Substance Abuse Treatment) are devoted to program development and evaluation. A quick glance at their website (www.samhsa.gov) reveals their interests in assessing a variety of programs from jail diversion to suicide prevention. The Centers for Disease Control and Prevention (CDC), with a budget of $7 billion, directs most of its funding to organizations rather than individuals. CDC-funded studies run the gamut from infectious disease surveillance to suicide prevention to cancer control (see www.cdc.gov for more information).

Community-based participatory research (CBPR) has attracted the interest of NIH as well as smaller private foundations. Areas of particular interest and suitability include HIV/AIDS prevention, cancer prevention and control, nutrition, and environmental contamination. The vanguard in CBPR work at NIH has been the National Institute for Environmental Health Sciences (NIEHS). In 1994, an Environmental Justice and CBPR program was initiated to foster community collaboration in research, also partnering with the Environmental Protection Agency (EPA) and the National Institute for Occupational Safety and Health (NIOSH). For more information, go to www.niehs.nih.gov/research/supported/pro grams/justice/.

Most funding initiatives are time-limited, and the reader is advised to periodically check the relevant websites for updates and new funding announcements.

Getting Past the Catch-22

Seasoned researchers usually do better at obtaining external funding than their less experienced counterparts (although seniority is no guarantee of success). Two simple reasons account for this. First is the Catch-22 that comes when review committees give higher ratings to experienced, proven researchers (on the reasonable assumption that their qualifications will enhance the study's probability of success). Second, mature researchers are usually better able to put together a credible, strong proposal drawing on their experience and knowledge of what it takes. This advantage affects qualitative and mixed methods investigators in particular since the researcher-as-instrument aspect of their work favors those who are highly qualified "instruments."

How does a novice overcome these drawbacks? New investigators can succeed by taking a few strategically planned actions. First, they can seek the mentorship of senior researchers in their area who have successful funding track records. If possible, one's mentors are included in the proposal as a coinvestigator, consultant, and so on. Second, they should seek out successful proposals in their areas of interest and emulate them. There are many things that can be learned this way, including how the "argument" is made (see Box A.1 for an example), how much emphasis to place on methods, what a budget should look like, how to handle ethical issues, proper use of terminology, and so forth. Researchers can go to the NIH RePORT system (Research Portfolio Online Reporting Tools) at http:// projectreporter.nih.gov/reporter.cfm to examine abstracts from successfully funded proposals to get both inspiration and information.

Box A.1   Making a Compelling Argument: Rhetoric and Reason

Proposals seeking funding must address a huge "so what?" question designed to ensure that funds are expended wisely. Here are the opening paragraphs of the grant proposal I submitted to the National Institute of Mental Health in 2004. I am grateful to my erudite coinvestigator, Dr. Kim Hopper, for supplying most of the compelling rhetoric embedded in this excerpt:

> Psychiatrically disabled homeless adults lead complex, troubled lives struggling to meet basic survival needs and cope with serious mental illness. Their lives often complicated by substance abuse, such individuals present a standing challenge to a resource-strapped service system designed with more stable clients, more discretely packaged needs, and more predictable trajectories of service use in mind. Patient-centered care is problematic, seeming to pit wary veterans of street and shelter life against systems concerned about scarce resources and public safety. In community debates, these apparently conflicting priorities are often portrayed as weary providers confronted by recalcitrant men and women who seem to prefer the dangerous freedom of street life to the security, structure, and self-discipline of rehabilitation.

(Continued)

(Continued)

> While doubtless oversimplified, it is difficult to fault this portrait since available research has brought precision at the cost of narrowed scope, i.e., it has provided a "top-down" perspective on the gap between need and use of services among psychiatrically disabled homeless adults. Studies have been *thorough* in measuring the prevalence of problems and *focused* on testing interventions for their resolution, but they have also been partial in perspective. In this contested arena of competing interests, *the service user's perspective remains poorly documented and understood.*

Commentary: Notice a few things about these two paragraphs: (1) Italics are used judiciously for emphasis (not recommended for dissertations and scholarly reports); (2) the argument is made for conducting a qualitative study, but its rhetorical power depends on the sad realities of life for homeless mentally ill adults; (3) the paragraphs are densely packed and touch on several key issues— comorbid substance abuse, public safety concerns, the lack of "fit" between the service system and consumers, and the limitations of extant research; (4) this sets the stage for the study that is specified in greater detail in the proposal. In other words, rhetoric must sooner or later be linked to substance.

Setting the Stage

Resources and Environment: The Importance of Research Infrastructure(s)

Virtually every funder requires assurances that the research environment is supportive to the study; that is, the necessary resources ranging from libraries to computers are available. This speaks to a larger "backstage" issue in grant getting: the wide variation in supportive infrastructure at institutions where researchers work. Colleges and universities with heavy teaching loads and limited support staff are vastly different from large research-intensive universities that derive a major source of revenue from the overhead generated by external funding. For the latter, there is a reasonable expectation of sufficient space (laboratories, interviewing suites, computer terminals, staff offices) and resources (statistical software, computer servers with large storage capacity, clerical assistance) to sustain intensive research endeavors.

Even further backstage are infrastructure supports that can make the researcher's ability to obtain funding far easier. These include a formal mentoring system; an IRB (institutional review board) liaison; and funds for pilot studies, methods consultants, cross-language translation, and training workshops. A vibrant, productive research office would bring in outside presenters and experts to supplement in-house expertise. It might sponsor regular lectures and writing groups. Staff would be available to prepare ancillary portions of grant applications such as the budget pages, budget justification, and IRB applications. They would oversee collecting and assembling bio-sketches of key personnel and support letters from sites. At the other end of the process, support staff would assist in dissemination of the findings through website postings, newsletters, press releases, policy briefs, and so on.

As mentioned earlier in this book, qualitative studies are low-tech and inexpensive when compared to a randomized trial. However, they still require resources and are labor-intensive. Infrastructure supports associated with these methods include (in addition to the above) transcriptionists, community liaisons (especially for CBPR), travel to and from study sites for preliminary planning, and QDA software.

Working With Communities and Other Study Settings

For site-specific studies, the researcher needs to have good working relationships for a variety of reasons, not least of which is to ensure that necessary forms of cooperation will be forthcoming. Cooperation can range from posting a recruitment flyer to allowing access to an agency or clinic's operations to the full-bore partnerships characteristic of CBPR. Sampling needs should be met within a reasonable time period and verified by the cooperating sites if they are to be involved. Appending support letters to the grant proposal is an important step.

The principal investigator may want to establish consortium agreements among sites if a significant level of involvement is being sought. A memorandum of understanding (MOU) is strongly advised when there are multiple stakeholders involved in the study who must enact multiple roles. The MOU helps prevent misunderstandings by clarifying these roles and laying the groundwork for the cooperation needed to carry out the study. Pilot or preliminary study findings enhance confidence in the researcher's commitment and the study's feasibility. The more this preparatory work can be incorporated into the proposal, the better.

Finally, although it may seem obvious, the researcher should corral all necessary proposal materials as early as possible. These typically include budget information, support letters, appendices, departmental approval letters, bio-sketches of key personnel, and so forth. Waiting until the last minute will add enormous strain to the nail-biting process of assembling all of the proposal's parts and getting them in on time.

Questions From Reviewers Regarding Qualitative Methods Proposals

A qualitative methods proposal has a better chance than ever before, but it is still likely to arouse methodological concerns (Munhall, 1994; Ungar, 2006). Here, more than ever, transparency and specificity are needed.

The review of grant proposals varies somewhat depending on the funding source (foundation, government, private donor, institutional funds, etc.), but it invariably involves evaluating the study's overall significance, its methods, and its fit with the funding organization's mission. Typically, a panel of experienced researchers reviews and rates the proposals, and meets to discuss their merits and recommend those deemed worthy of funding. Positive peer reviews are necessary but not always sufficient since funding may also depend upon budgetary allowances and, at times, other expert opinions.

The following are some of the questions reviewers might put to the proposal (and to the researcher if she were present in the room):

- How can we be sure that the findings will justify the amount of money requested?
- Do the principal investigator and the research team have enough experience to make this study a success?
- Is this study really filling a gap in knowledge?
- Is this study innovative?
- Are there ethical problems created by asking people sensitive questions or observing them in situ?
- Is this study feasible given the time and money being requested?
- How do we know that the methods are rigorous?
- Is the sampling strategy biased?
- Do the study findings have implications for practice/policy/future research?
- Will the findings be generalizable?
- Will this study contribute to theory development?
- Qualitative studies seem to rely more on faith in the researcher than in the methods. Does this proposal counteract this impression?

The researcher would do well to anticipate and answer these questions in the proposal. Most if not all of the answers can be found elsewhere in this book. Box A.2 gives a detailed description of how reviews of grant proposals take place at the NIH, a process that is similar to that of other funding venues.

Box A.2   The Review Process at the National Institutes of Health (NIH)

Primary advantages to NIH funding are the ample budgets that are possible and the high rates of indirect costs, or the percentage allocated to the researcher's institution to cover facilities and administration expenses (often well over 50%). By comparison, private foundations usually fund at lower levels and pay indirect costs at lower rates (or not at all). Among the 27 institutes and centers at the NIH, a few are the most receptive to qualitative and mixed methods: NIMH (National Institute of Mental Health), NIDA (National Institute on Drug Abuse), NCI (National Cancer Institute), NICHD (National Institute on Child Health and Development), NIEHS (National Institute for Environmental and Health Sciences), and NINR (National Institute of Nursing Research). Annual budgets differ (NINR's budget is a tiny fraction of NCI's), and review panels across the institutes vary in their expectations and rigor.

Although the NIH sometimes makes minor changes in its extramural funding procedures, the process unfolds in a predictable, if poorly understood, fashion. After the proposal has been submitted electronically, it is usually sent to the CSR (Center for Scientific Review) where an administrator identifies the correct institute and study section and assigns it to the reviewers (at least one of whom ideally has qualitative methods expertise). The reviewers consider strengths and weaknesses along the following parameters: overall impact/priority, significance (Why is this study needed and important?), innovation (Does the study use novel approaches and ideas?), investigators (Do the investigators have the necessary qualifications for the study?), approach (What are the study's methods, are they appropriate to the aims, and how rigorous are they?), and environment (Does the home institution offer an appropriate platform for the study?). Additional review criteria include protection of human subjects; inclusion of women, minorities, and children (a federal requirement unless a convincing counterargument is made); and budget (Is the proposed budget sufficient to carry out the study but not excessive or inappropriate?).

(Continued)

(Continued)

Reviewers, who receive online access to the proposals around 6 weeks in advance of the panel meeting, are expected to submit their critiques and a suggested score on a secure Internet site before the meeting. Increasingly, reviewers may be asked to attend via speakerphone to save costs, but most still attend in person and convene at a hotel near NIH headquarters in Maryland. During or right before the meeting, the aggregate scores are reviewed, and typically the bottom 50% of the proposals are recommended for tabling from full-panel discussion (a higher percentage may be tabled if funding is limited). Submitters not given panel review still receive the reviewers' written critiques along with their "unscored" verdict. The scoring range is from 1.0 (exceptional, virtually flawless) to 9.0 (poor, with few strengths and numerous major weaknesses).

For the fortunate upper tier of proposals, an intense discussion takes place in which the assigned reviewers present their critiques amidst panel discussion of the proposal's merits. Each proposal is ultimately given a score by all members of the panel (influenced no doubt by the assigned reviewers' comments), and the aggregate score and a percentile ranking is posted on the NIH Commons website (https://commons.era.nih.gov/commons/) where researchers will have enrolled previously. The full critique, or Summary Statement, is posted on the Commons website 4–6 weeks after the meeting. Although the cut-point for funding is unfortunately sliding lower (the top 20% of proposals used to be assured of success), a score under 3.0 and/or a percentile ranking of 15 or lower gives reason for hope. The actual funding decision is made by the institute's council (a group of eminent researchers), who is charged with enacting that institute's funding priorities. It is the rare council, however, that stands in the way of an excellent score.

The majority of proposals to NIH are not funded on the first round, and researchers have only one additional opportunity to revise and resubmit. The revision is expected to follow the previous critique closely and highlight changes made. Contacts with one's program officer can help immeasurably in deciphering the review and deciding on revisions.

The following are a few additional pointers:

- Go to http://cms.csr.nih.gov/ResourcesforApplicants/ for more information.
- Contact the appropriate institute program officer in advance and get his or her advice on shaping the proposal. Keep in mind, however, that

program officers do not make funding decisions. They must sit silently while the panel does its work.

- Attach a cover letter to ensure that your proposal goes to the right review committee. Many a researcher has taken this for granted and then found the proposal sent to a committee with little understanding or sympathy for the topic and methods.
- Don't give up—even the most senior researchers get rejected and the most junior researchers get funded.

Budgeting Time and Resources

Forecasting the required amount of time and resources—and their associated costs—imposes a degree of precision all too rare in qualitative inquiry. Yet formulas can be calculated based on desired sample sizes and generally known information for the time it takes to conduct and transcribe interviews, equipment and software costs, incentive payments, and so forth. Ultimately, research budgets must reflect the study's proposed reach and available resources.

Budget categories include *personnel salaries and fringe benefits* (investigators, interviewers, research assistants, etc.), *equipment* (audio recorders, laptops for field notes, etc.), *research supplies* (software, batteries, CD-ROMs, flash memory drives, etc.), *transportation costs* (subway/bus fares), *participant incentives and services* (transcription, expert consultant fees), and *travel to conferences* for presentations. *Site fees* may be paid to compensate staff for assistance in recruitment and data collection. If allowed, *indirect costs* (also called overhead) are computed as a percentage of the direct costs to pay for office rent, clerical help, utilities, and so on. Allocations within and across these categories must reflect a realistic appraisal of what is needed (i.e., neither wildly inflated nor unrealistically underbudgeted). Researchers should adhere to extant norms about incentive payments, consultant pay rates, and transcription costs. Budgeting for interviews starts from the ground up. As a hypothetical example, assume that the study involves two 90-minute interviews with 50 participants and transcription costs are $15 an hour. This amounts to 100 interviews times 1.5 hours or 150 hours of audio needing transcription. Because the ratio of recording hours to transcription hours is anywhere from 1 to 3 to 1 to 8, it would be reasonable to allocate funds for 150 (recording) hours times 5 (transcription) hours, or 750 hours total for transcription time.

At a rate of $15 per hour, this equals $11,250 for transcription. Incentives at $25 per interview (50 participants, each having two interviews) equals $2,500, and so forth.

These calculations should be fully explained and rationalized in the *budget justification*. As such, they vividly illustrate the backstage labors involved in qualitative studies and offer a rationale for generously funding even a "small sample" study. Indeed, the budget justification can help a proposal considerably by demonstrating how intense and time-consuming rigorous qualitative studies can be.

Twenty Tips for Writing the Proposal

The following guidelines or tips can be turned into a handy checklist for planning and writing the proposal.

1. Start with a compelling, unanswered study question(s) that will impress the reviewers.

2. Make sure the study begins with specific aims and research questions that present a clear road map for the study.

3. Write a concise but comprehensive abstract. (Remember that this may be the only description of your study widely disseminated later on.)

4. Include a rationale for use of qualitative or mixed methods and their requisite strengths.

5. Ground the study in a coherent, strong theoretical framework. Qualitative studies are not considered exempt from this expectation, but their inductive nature should be highlighted and the various theoretical "lenses" presented with this caveat.

6. Make sure that ethical guidelines are followed and all potential threats to human subjects are minimized or eliminated.

7. If the budget allows, include expert consultants who can provide guidance on methods or other specialized study needs.

8. Be direct and explicit about research design, including an explanation for why qualitative designs need to be flexible and iterative. For mixed methods studies, address how the two "sides" will be dealt with, whether that means triangulation, integration, and so on.

9. Describe in detail the sampling and recruitment plans.

10. Build in a pilot study to ensure that protocols get a trial run-through.

11. Describe procedures for retaining study participants (contact information, payment of incentives, etc.). This is critical for longitudinal designs.

12. Structure the data analysis section around each specific aim or study goal and describe step-by-step how the analyses will be carried out.

13. Include in each data analysis section a subsection titled "Strategies for Rigor" and indicate which will be used (as appropriate).

14. Include a table in the proposal with some version of the following columns: Specific Aims (or Research Questions), Sample Size and Source, Sampling Criteria and Recruitment, Sources of Data, Type of Data Analysis, Time Frame. Reading across, each row is a specific aim followed by its requisite information.

15. Include a timeline showing the length of the study (in months) on the x-axis and each task stacked up along the y-axis. Lines and arrows are used to show each task's beginning and ending point.

16. If appropriate (and this is often the case), build a community advisory board (CAB) into the proposal. CABs provide valuable input and are an indication that the study is (and will be) responsive.

17. Make sure the budget is reasonable but not skimpy—feasibility and credibility matter.

18. Observe page limitations, font sizes, and margins carefully. Ignoring these might result in a returned (or discarded) proposal.

19. If appropriate, include plans for dissemination of the study findings. Funders might want to be a part of this process to varying degrees, but all have a vested interest in seeing the study's conclusions influencing practice, policy, and future research. Professional conferences and other presentation venues are excellent opportunities to disseminate, but the ultimate impact comes from publication in peer-reviewed, respected outlets.

20. Be patient and prepared to submit again (or somewhere else)!

Additional Readings and Web Resources

Locke L., Spirduso, W., & Silverman, S. (Eds.). (2007). *Proposals that work: A guide for planning dissertations and grant proposals* (5th ed.). Thousand Oaks, CA: Sage.

Morse, J. M. (1994). Designing funded qualitative research. In N. K. Denzin & Y. S. Lincoln (Eds.), *Handbook of qualitative research* (pp. 220–235). Thousand Oaks, CA: Sage.

Munhall, P. L. (1994). *Qualitative research proposals and reports: A guide.* New York: National League for Nursing Press.

National Institutes of Health. (1999). *Qualitative methods in health research: Opportunities and considerations in application and review.* Bethesda, MD: Office of Behavioral and Social Science Research (OBSSR). Available at http://obssr.od.nih.gov/pdf/Qualitative.PDF

Ungar, M. (2006). "Too ambitious": What happens when funders misunderstand the strength of qualitative research design. *Qualitative Social Work, 5*(2), 261–277.

Yang, O. O. (2007). *Guide to effective grant writing: How to write an effective NIH grant application.* New York: Springer.

Information on Federal Funding Opportunities

In the United States:

http://www.grants.gov (CDC)
http://grants.nih.gov/grants/oer.htm (NIH)
http://obssr.od.nih.gov/pdf/Qualitative.PDF (NIH guide for writing and submitting qualitative proposals)
http://www.samhsa.gov/grants/ (Substance Abuse and Mental Health Services Administration)
http://www.nsf.gov (National Science Foundation)
http://phpartners.org/grants.html (Public Health Grant Information)
http://projectreporter.nih.gov/reporter.cfm (Abstracts of NIH-funded projects)

In Canada:

http://www.cihr-irsc.gc.ca/ (Canadian Institutes of Health Research)

In the United Kingdom:

http://www.nihr.ac.uk/research/Pages/default.aspx (National Institute for Health Research)

In Australia:

http://www.nhmrc.gov.au/ (National Health and Medical Research Council)

In New Zealand:

http://www.frst.govt.nz/ (Foundation for Research, Science and Technology)

References

Abbott, A. (1997). Of time and space: The contemporary relevance of the Chicago School. *Social Forces, 75*(4), 1145–1182.

Agar, M. H. (1980). *The professional stranger: An informal introduction to ethnography.* New York: Academic Press.

Agar, M. H. (1991). The right brain strikes back. In N. G. Fielding & R. M. Lee (Eds.), *Using computers in qualitative research* (pp. 181–194). Newbury Park, CA: Sage.

Agar, M. H., & MacDonald, J. (1995). Focus groups and ethnography. *Human Organization, 54*(1), 78–86.

Allison, K. R., & Rootman, I. (1996). Scientific rigor and community participation in health promotion research: Are they compatible? *Health Promotion International, 11*(4), 333–340.

Altheide, D. L., & Johnson, J. M. (1994). Criteria for assessing interpretive validity in qualitative research. In N. K. Denzin & Y. S. Lincoln (Eds.), *Handbook of qualitative research* (pp. 485–499). Thousand Oaks, CA: Sage.

Anfara, V. A., & Mertz, N. T. (Eds.). (2006). *Theoretical frameworks in qualitative research.* Thousand Oaks, CA: Sage.

Annells, M. (1996). Grounded theory method: Philosophical perspectives, paradigm of research, and postmodernism. *Qualitative Health Research, 6*(3), 379–393.

Annells, M. (2006). Triangulation of qualitative approaches: Phenomenology and grounded theory. *Journal of Advanced Nursing, 56*(1), 55–61.

Atkinson, J. M., & Heritage, J. (Eds.). (1984). *Structure of social action: Studies in conversation analysis.* Cambridge, UK: Cambridge University Press.

Atkinson, P. (1997). Narrative turn or blind alley? *Qualitative Health Research, 7*(3), 325–344.

Atkinson, P. (2005, September). Qualitative research—Unity and diversity [25 paragraphs]. *Forum Qualitative Sozialforschung/Forum: Qualitative Social Research, 6*(3), Article 26. Available at http://www.qualitative-research.net/index.php/fqs/article/view/4/9

Atkinson, P., & Silverman, D. (1997). Kundera's immortality: The interview society and the invention of the self. *Qualitative Inquiry, 3,* 304–325.

Baker, C., Wuest, J., & Stern, P. N. (1992). Method slurring: The grounded theory/phenomenology example. *Journal of Advanced Nursing, 17*, 1335–1360.

Barkin, S., Ryan, G., & Gelberg, L. (1999). What pediatricians can do to further violence prevention: A qualitative study. *Injury Prevention, 5*, 53–58.

Baum, F. (1996). Researching public health: Behind the qualitative–quantitative methodological debate. *Social Science & Medicine, 40*(4), 459–468.

Beck, C. T. (1993). Teetering on the edge: A substantive theory of postpartum depression. *Nursing Research, 42*(1), 42–50.

Beck, C. T. (2005). Benefits of participating in Internet interviews: Women helping women. *Qualitative Health Research, 15*(3), 411–422.

Becker, H. (1996). The epistemology of qualitative research. In R. Jessor, A. Colby, & R. Schweder (Eds.), *Ethnography and human development* (pp. 53–72). Chicago: University of Chicago Press.

Beebe, J. (2002). *Rapid assessment process.* Lanham, MD: AltaMira Press.

Benner, P. (Ed.). (1994). *Interpretive phenomenology: Embodiment, caring, and ethics in health and illness.* Thousand Oaks, CA: Sage.

Berelson, B. (1952). *Content analysis in communication research.* Glencoe, IL: The Free Press.

Berger, P., & Luckmann, T. (1967). *The social construction of reality.* New York: Doubleday.

Bloor, M. (1997). Techniques of validation in qualitative research: A critical commentary. In G. Miller & R. Dingwall (Eds.), *Context and method in qualitative research* (pp. 37–50). London: Sage.

Boeri, M. W. (2004). "Hell, I'm an addict, but I ain't no Junkie": An ethnographic analysis of aging heroin users. *Human Organization, 63*(2), 236–246.

Bogdan, R. C., & Taylor, S. J. (1975). *Introduction to qualitative research.* New York: Wiley.

Bohm, A. (2004). Theoretical coding: Text analysis in grounded theory. In U. Flick, E. von Kardorff, & I. Steinke (Eds.), *A companion to qualitative research* (pp. 270–275). London: Sage.

Bowen, G. A. (2006). Grounded theory and sensitizing concepts. *International Journal of Qualitative Methods, 5*(3), Article 2.

Bowen, G. A. (2008). Naturalistic inquiry and the saturation concept: A research note. *Qualitative Research, 8*, 137–152.

Boyatzis, R. E. (1998). *Transforming qualitative information: Thematic analysis and code development.* Thousand Oaks, CA: Sage.

Bozeman, B., Slade, C., & Hirsch, P. (2009). Understanding bureaucracy in health science ethics: Toward a better institutional review board. *American Journal of Public Health, 99*(9), 1549–1556.

Bradley, E. H., Curry, L. A., & Devers, K. J. (2007). Qualitative data analysis for health services research: Developing taxonomy, themes, and theory. *Health Services Research, 42*(4), 1758–1772.

Bradshaw, T. K. (1999). Communities not fazed: Why military base closures may not be catastrophic. *Journal of American Planning Association, 65*, 193–206.

Bryman, A. (2006). Integrating quantitative and qualitative research: How is it done? *Qualitative Research, 6*(1), 97–113.

Caelli, K., Ray, L., & Mill, J. (2003). "Clear as mud": Toward greater clarity in generic qualitative research. *International Journal of Qualitative Methods, 2*(2).

Campbell, D. T. (1979). Degrees of freedom and the case study. In T. D. Cook & C. S. Reichart (Eds.), *Qualitative and quantitative methods in evaluation research* (pp. 49–67). Beverly Hills, CA: Sage.

Campbell, D. T., & Stanley, J. C. (1963). *Experimental and quasi-experimental designs for research.* Boston: Houghton Mifflin.

Campbell, R., & Arens, C. E. (1998). Innovative community services for rape victims: An application of multiple case study methodology. *American Journal of Community Psychology, 26*(4), 537–571.

Caracelli, V. J., & Greene, J. C. (1997). Crafting mixed-methods evaluations designs. In J. C. Greene & V. J. Caracelli (Eds.), *Advances in mixed-method evaluation: The challenges and benefits of integrating diverse paradigms* (*New Directions for Evaluation*, No. 74, pp. 19–32). San Francisco: Jossey-Bass.

Carlson, E. D., Engebretson, J., & Chamberlain, R. M. (2006). Photovoice as a social process of critical consciousness. *Qualitative Health Research, 16*(6), 836–852.

Cashman, S. B., Adeky, S., Allen, A. J., Corburn, J., Israel, B. A., Montano, J., et al. (2008). The power and the promise: Working with communities to analyze data, interpret findings, and get to outcomes. *American Journal of Public Health, 98*(8), 1407–1417.

Castro, A., & Farmer, P. (2005). Understanding and addressing AIDS-related stigma: From anthropological theory to clinical practice in Haiti. *American Journal of Public Health, 95*(1), 53–59.

Chambers, E. (2000). Applied ethnography. In N. K. Denzin & Y. S. Lincoln (Eds.), *Handbook of qualitative research* (pp. 851–869, 2nd ed.). Thousand Oaks, CA: Sage.

Charmaz, K. (2006). *Constructing grounded theory.* Thousand Oaks, CA: Sage.

Chen, P. G., Diaz, N., Lucas, G., & Rosenthal, M. S. (2010). Dissemination of results in community-based participatory research. *American Journal of Preventive Medicine, 39*(4), 372–378.

Cherryholmes, C. H. (1992). Notes on pragmatism and scientific realism. *Educational Researcher, 14*, 13–17.

Chiovitti, R. F., & Piran, N. (2003). Rigour and grounded theory research. *Journal of Advanced Nursing, 44*(4), 427–435.

Christians, C. G. (2000). Ethics and politics in qualitative research. In N. K. Denzin & Y. S. Lincoln (Eds.), *Handbook of qualitative research* (pp. 133–155, 2nd ed.). Thousand Oaks, CA: Sage.

Chung, K., & Lounsbury, D. (2006). The role of power, process, and relationships in participatory research for statewide HIV/AIDS programming. *Social Science & Medicine, 63*(8), 2129–2140.

Cifuentes, E., Alamo, U., Kendall, T., Brunkard, J., & Scrimshaw, S. (2006). Rapid assessment procedures in environmental sanitation research. *Canadian Journal of Public Health, 97*(1), 24–28.

Clarke, A. (2005). *Situational analysis: Grounded theory after the postmodern turn.* Thousand Oaks, CA: Sage.

Clifford, J., & Marcus, G. E. (Eds.). (1986). *Writing culture: The poetics and politics of ethnography.* Berkeley: University of California Press.

Cochran, P. L., Marshall, C. A., Garcia-Downing, C., Kendall, E., Cook, D., McCubbin, L., et al. (2008). Indigenous ways of knowing: Implications for participatory research and community. *American Journal of Public Health, 98*(1), 22–27.

Coffey, A., & Atkinson, P. (1996). *Making sense of qualitative data.* Thousand Oaks, CA: Sage.

Colaizzi, P. F. (1978). Psychological research as the phenomenologist views it. In R. Valle & M. King (Eds.), *Existential-phenomenological alternatives for psychology* (pp. 48–71). New York: Oxford University Press.

Cook, T. D., & Campbell, D. T. (1979). *Quasi-experimentation: Design and analysis issues for field settings.* Boston: Houghton Mifflin.

Cook, T. D., & Reichardt, C. S. (Eds.). (1979). *Qualitative and quantitative methods in evaluation* research. Beverly Hills, CA: Sage.

Cooney, K. (2006). Mothers first, not work first: Listening to welfare clients in job training. *Qualitative Social Work, 5*(2), 217–235.

Cooper, C. M., & Yarbrough, S. P. (2010, May). Tell me—show me: Using combined focus group and photovoice methods to gain understanding of health issues in rural Guatemala. *Qualitative Health Research, 20*(5), 644–653.

Cornish, F., & Ghosh, R. (2007). The necessary contradictions of community-led health promotion: A case study of HIV prevention in an Indian red light district. *Social Science & Medicine, 64*(2), 496–507.

Cornwall, A., & Jewkes, R. (1995). What is participatory research? *Social Science & Medicine, 41*(12), 1667–1676.

Correll, S. (1995). The ethnography of an electronic bar: The lesbian café. *Journal of Contemporary Ethnography, 24*(3), 270–294.

Crabtree, B. F., & Miller, W. L. (1999). *Doing qualitative research* (2nd ed.). Thousand Oaks, CA: Sage.

Creswell, J. W. (2003). *Research design: Qualitative, quantitative, and mixed methods approaches* (2nd ed.). Thousand Oaks, CA: Sage.

Creswell, J. W. (2007). *Qualitative inquiry and research design* (2nd ed.). Thousand Oaks, CA: Sage.

Creswell, J. W., & Plano Clark, V. (2010). *Designing and conducting mixed methods research* (2nd ed.). Thousand Oaks, CA: Sage.

Czarniawska, B. (2004). *Narratives in social science research.* Thousand Oaks, CA: Sage.

Czymoniewicz-Klippel, M. T., Brijnath, B., & Crockett, B. (2010, June). Ethics and the promotion of inclusiveness within qualitative research: Case examples from Asia and the Pacific. *Qualitative Inquiry 16*(5), 332–341.

Daly, J. (2009). Qualitative methods and the curse of the illustrative quotation. *Australian and New Zealand Journal of Public Health, 33*(5), 405–406.

Davis, M., Rhodes, T., & Martin, A. (2004). Preventing hepatitis C: Common sense, the bug, and other perspectives from the risk narratives of people who inject drugs. *Social Science & Medicine, 59*(9), 1807–1818.

DeMarco, R., Carswell, K., Hornowski, K., & Snider, L. (2005). *Conducting a participatory situation analysis of orphans and vulnerable children affected by HIV/AIDS: Guidelines and tools.* Research Triangle Park, NC: Family Health International. Available online at http://www.fhi.org/en/HIVAIDS/pub/guide/ovcguide.htm

Denzin, N. K. (1978). *The research act: A theoretical introduction to sociological methods* (2nd ed.). New York: McGraw-Hill.

Denzin, N. K. (1989). *Interpretive interactionism.* Newbury Park, CA: Sage.

Denzin, N. K. (1994). The art and politics of interpretation. In N. K. Denzin & Y. S. Lincoln (Eds.), *Handbook of qualitative research* (pp. 500–515). Thousand Oaks, CA: Sage.

Denzin, N. K., & Lincoln, Y. S. (Eds.). (1994). *Handbook of qualitative research.* Thousand Oaks, CA: Sage.

Denzin, N. K., & Lincoln, Y. S. (Eds.). (2000). *Handbook of qualitative research* (2nd ed.). Thousand Oaks, CA: Sage.

Denzin, N. K., & Lincoln, Y. S. (Eds.). (2005). *The SAGE handbook of qualitative research* (3rd ed.). Thousand Oaks, CA: Sage.

DeSilva, M. J., Harpham, T., Tuan, T., Bartolini, R., Penny, M. E., & Huttly, S. R. (2006). Psychometric and cognitive validation of a social capital measurement tool in Peru and Vietnam. *Social Science & Medicine, 62,* 941–953.

Dick, H. P. (2006). What to do with "I don't know": Elicitation in ethnographic and survey interviews. *Qualitative Sociology, 29*(1), 87–102.

Dickson-Swift, V., James, E. L., Kippen, S., & Liamputtong, P. (2007). Doing sensitive research: What challenges do qualitative researchers face? *Qualitative Research, 7*(3), 327–353.

Dixon-Woods, M., Booth, A., & Sutton, A. J. (2007). Synthesizing qualitative research: A review of published reports. *Qualitative Research, 7*(3), 375–422.

Dixon-Woods, M., & Fitzpatrick, R. (2001). Qualitative research in systematic reviews. *British Medical Journal, 323,* 65–66.

Donmoyer, R. (1990). Generalizability and the single-case study. In E. W. Eisner & A. Peshkin (Eds.), *Qualitative inquiry in education: The continuing debate* (pp. 175–200). New York: Teachers College Press.

Drake, R. E., Bebout, R. R., Quimby, E., Teague, G. B., Harris, M., & Roach, J. P. (1993). Process evaluation in the Washington, D.C., Dual Diagnosis Project. *Alcoholism Treatment Quarterly, 10,* 113–124.

Duneier, M. (1999). *Sidewalk*. New York: Farrar, Straus & Giroux.

Dupuis, A., & Thorns, D. C. (1998). Home, home ownership, and the search for ontological security. *The Sociological Review, 46*(1), 24–47.

Ellis, C., & Bochner, A. P. (2000). Autoethnography, personal narrative, reflexivity: Researcher as subject. In N. K. Denzin & Y. S. Lincoln (Eds.), *Handbook of qualitative research* (2nd ed., pp. 733–768). Thousand Oaks, CA: Sage.

Ellis, C., & Flaherty, M. G. (1992). An agenda for the interpretation of lived experience. In E. Ellis & M. G. Flaherty (Eds.), *Investigating subjectivity: Research on lived experience* (pp. 1–16). Newbury Park, CA: Sage.

Ely, M., Anzul, M., Friedman, T., Garner, D., & Steinmetz, A. M. (1991). *Doing qualitative research: Circles within circles*. London: Falmer Press.

Emerson, R. (2001). *Contemporary field research: Perspectives and formulations*. Long Grove, IL: Waveland Press.

Emerson, R. M., Fretz, R. I., & Shaw, L. L. (1995). *Writing ethnographic fieldnotes*. Chicago: University of Chicago Press.

Eng, E., Moore, K. S., Rhodes, S. D., Griffith, D. M., Allison, L. L., Shirah, K., et al. (2005). Insiders and outsiders assess who is "the community." In B. A. Israel, E. Eng, A. J. Schulz, & E. A. Parker (Eds.), *Methods in community-based participatory research for health* (pp. 77–100). San Francisco: Jossey-Bass.

Erickson, F. (1986). Qualitative methods in research on teaching. In M. C. Wittrock (Ed.), *Handbook of research on teaching* (3rd ed., pp. 119–161). New York: Macmillan.

Ericsson, C. (2000). Learning and knowledge production for public health: A review of approaches in evidence-based public health. *Scandinavian Journal of Public Health, 28*, 298–308.

Esposito, N. (2001). From meaning to meaning: The influence of translation techniques on non-English focus group research. *Qualitative Health Research, 11*(4), 568–579.

Estroff, S. (1981). *Making it crazy*. Berkeley: University of California Press.

Fals-Borda, O. (Ed.). (1998). *People's participation: Challenges ahead*. New York: Apex.

Fals-Borda, O., & Rahman, M. A. (Eds.). (1991). *Action and knowledge: Breaking the monopoly with participatory action research*. New York: Intermediate Technology/Apex.

Faltermaier, T. (1997). Why public health research needs qualitative approaches: Subjects and methods in change. *The European Journal of Public Health, 7*(4), 357–363.

Farnell, B., & Graham, L. R. (2000). Discourse-centered methods. In H. R. Bernard (Ed.), *Handbook of methods in cultural anthropology* (pp. 411–454). Walnut Creek, CA: AltaMira Press.

Feagin, J. R., Orum, A. M., & Sjoberg, G. (Eds.). (1991). *A case for the case study*. Chapel Hill: University of North Carolina Press.

Felton, B. J. (2005). Defining location in the mental health system: A case study of a consumer-run agency. *American Journal of Community Psychology, 36*, 373–386.

Fereday, J., & Muir-Cochrane, E. (2006). Demonstrating rigor using thematic analysis: A hybrid approach of inductive and deductive coding and theme development. *International Journal of Qualitative Methods, 5*(1), Article 1.

Fetterman, D. M. (1989). *Ethnography: Step by step.* Newbury Park, CA: Sage.

Fine, G. A., & Martin, D. D. (1990). A partisan view: Sarcasm, satire, and irony as voices in Erving Goffman's *Asylums. Journal of Contemporary Ethnography, 19,* 89–115.

Flaherty, M. G. (2002). The "crisis" in representation: Reflections and assessments. *Journal of Contemporary Ethnography, 31*(4), 508–516.

Flick, U. (2004). Triangulation in qualitative research. In U. Flick, E. von Kardorff, & I. Steinke (Eds.), *A companion to qualitative research* (pp. 178–183). London: Sage.

Flick, U., von Kardorff, E., & Steinke, I. (Eds.). (2004). *A companion to qualitative research.* London: Sage.

Flicker, S., Travers, R., Guta, A., McDonald, S., & Meagher, A. (2007). Ethical dilemmas in community-based participatory research: Recommendations for institutional review boards. *Journal of Urban Health, 84*(4), 478–493.

Flyvbjerg, B. (2006). Five misunderstandings about case-study research. *Qualitative Inquiry, 12*(2), 219–245.

Fonow, M. M., & Cook, J. A. (Eds.). (1991). *Beyond methodology: Feminist scholarship as lived research.* Bloomington: Indiana University Press.

Fontana, A., & Frey, J. H. (1994). Interviewing: The art of science. In N. K. Denzin & Y. S. Lincoln (Eds.), *Handbook of qualitative research* (pp. 361–376). Thousand Oaks, CA: Sage.

Ford, C. L., & Airhihenbuwa, C. O. (2010). The public health critical race methodology: Praxis for antiracism research. *Social Science and Medicine, 71,* 1390–1398.

Foster-Fishman, P., Berkowitz, S. L., Lounsbury, D. W., Jacobson, S., & Allen, N. (2001). Building collaborative capacity in community coalitions: A review and integrative framework. *American Journal of Community Psychology, 29*(2), 241–261.

Freeman, H. P. (2004). Poverty, culture, and social injustice: Determinants of cancer disparities. *A Cancer Journal for Clinicians, 54,* 72–77.

Freire, P. (1973). *Pedagogy of the oppressed.* New York: Soabury Press.

Freundlich, M., Avery, R. J., & Padgett, D. K. (2007). Care or scare: The safety of youth in congregate care in New York City. *Child Abuse & Neglect, 31*(2), 173–186.

Gair, S. (2002). In the thick of it: A reflective tale from an Australian social worker/qualitative researcher. *Qualitative Health Research, 12*(1), 130–139.

Gearing, R. E. (2004). Bracketing in research: A typology. *Qualitative Health Research, 14*(10), 1429–1452.

Gee, J. P. (2005). *An introduction to discourse analysis: Theory and method.* London: Routledge.

Geertz, C. (1973). *The interpretation of cultures: Selected essays.* New York: Basic Books.

Geertz, C. (1988). *Works and lives: The anthropologist as author.* Stanford, CA: Stanford University Press.

Gergen, M. M., & Gergen, K. J. (2000). Qualitative inquiry: Tensions and transformations. In N. K. Denzin & Y. S. Lincoln (Eds.), *Handbook of qualitative research* (2nd ed., pp. 1025–1046). Thousand Oaks, CA: Sage.

Giddens, A. (1990). *Consequences of modernity.* Oxford, UK: Polity Press.

Gioia, D. (2004). Mixed methods in a dissertation study. In D. K. Padgett (Ed.), *The qualitative research experience* (pp. 119–146). Belmont, CA: Thomson.

Giorgi, A. (Ed.). (1985). *Phenomenology and psychological research.* Pittsburgh, PA: Duquesne University Press.

Gipson, J. D., & Hindin, M. J. (2008). "Having another child would be a life or death situation for her": Understanding pregnancy termination among couples in rural Bangladesh. *American Journal of Public Health, 98*(10), 1827–1832.

Glaser, B. (1978). *Theoretical sensitivity.* Mill Valley, CA: The Sociology Press.

Glaser, B. G. (2002). Conceptualization: On theory and theorizing using grounded theory. *International Journal of Qualitative Methods, 1*(2), Article 3.

Glaser, B. G., & Strauss, A. L. (1967). *The discovery of grounded theory: Strategies for qualitative research.* Chicago: Aldine.

Goetz, J., & LeCompte, M. (1984). *Ethnography and qualitative design in educational research.* Orlando, FL: Academic Press.

Goffman, E. (1961). *Asylums: Essays on the social situation of mental patients and other inmates.* Garden City, NY: Basic Books.

Goleman, D. (2007, February 20). Flame first, think later: New clues to email misbehavior. *New York Times,* p. F5.

González-López, G. (2010). Ethnographic lessons: Researching incest in Mexican families. *Journal of Contemporary Ethnography, 39*(5), 569–581.

Gooden, R. J., & Winefield, H. R. (2007). Breast and prostate cancer online discussion boards: A thematic analysis of gender differences and similarities. *Journal of Health Psychology, 12*(1), 103–114.

Gotschi, E., Delve, R., & Freyer, B. (2009). Participatory photography as a qualitative approach to obtain insights into farmer groups. *Field Methods, 21*(3), 290–308.

Green, L. W., & Mercer, S. L. (2010, August 14). PRECEDE-PROCEED model: Encyclopedia of public health. *ENotes—Literature Study Guides, Lesson Plans, and More.* Available at http://www.enotes.com/public-health-encyclopedia/precede-proceed-model

Green, L. W., Ottoson, J. M., García, C., & Hiatt, R. A. (2009). Diffusion theory and knowledge dissemination, utilization, and integration in public health. *Annual Review of Public Health, 30*(1), 151–174.

Greene, J. C. (2000). Understanding social programs through evaluation. In N. K. Denzin & Y. S. Lincoln (Eds.), *Handbook of qualitative research* (2nd ed., pp. 981–1000). Thousand Oaks, CA: Sage.

Greene, J. C., & Caracelli, V. J. (Eds.). (1997). *Advances in mixed-method evaluation: The challenges and benefits of integrating diverse paradigms.* San Francisco: Jossey-Bass.

Gregory, D., Russell, C. K., & Phillips, L. R. (1997). Beyond textual perfection: Transcribers as vulnerable persons. *Qualitative Health Research, 7*(2), 294–300.

Griffin, L. J. (1993). Narrative, event-structure analysis, and causal interpretation in historical sociology. *American Journal of Sociology, 98,* 1094–1133.

Groenewald, T. (2004). A phenomenological research design illustrated. *International Journal of Qualitative Methods, 3*(1), Article 4.

Guba, E. G. (Ed.). (1990). *The paradigm dialog.* Newbury Park, CA: Sage.

Guba, E. G., & Lincoln, Y. S. (1981). *Effective evaluation.* San Francisco: Jossey-Bass.

Guba, E. G., & Lincoln, Y. S. (1989). *Fourth generation evaluation.* Newbury Park, CA: Sage.

Guba, E. G., & Lincoln, Y. S. (1994). Competing paradigms in qualitative research. In N. K. Denzin & Y. S. Lincoln (Eds.), *Handbook of qualitative research* (pp. 105–117). Thousand Oaks, CA: Sage.

Gubrium, J. F., & Holstein, J. A. (2000). Analyzing interpretive practice. In N. K. Denzin & Y. S. Lincoln (Eds.), *Handbook of qualitative research* (2nd ed., pp. 487–508). Thousand Oaks, CA: Sage.

Guest, G., Bunce, A., & Johnson, L. (2006). How many interviews are enough? An experiment with data saturation and variability. *Field Methods, 18*(1), 59–82.

Haase, J. E., & Myers, S. T. (1988). Reconciling paradigm assumptions of qualitative and quantitative research. *Western Journal of Nursing Research, 10,* 128–137.

Hall, A. L., & Rist, R. C. (1999). Integrating multiple qualitative research methods (or avoiding the precariousness of a one-legged stool). *Psychology & Marketing, 16,* 291–304.

Hall, C., & White, S. (2005). Looking inside professional practice. *Qualitative Social Work, 4*(4), 379–390.

Hamilton, R. J., & Bowers, B. J. (2006). Internet recruitment and email interviews in qualitative studies. *Qualitative Health Research, 16,* 821–835.

Harding, S. (1987). *Feminism and methodology.* Bloomington: Indiana University Press.

Hawkins, R. L., & Abrams, C. (2007). Disappearing acts: The social networks of formerly homeless individuals with co-occurring disorders. *Social Science & Medicine, 65,* 2031–2042.

Heckathorn, D. D. (1997). Respondent-driven sampling: A new approach to the study of hidden populations. *Social Problems, 44*(2), 174–199.

Hertz, R., & Imber, J. B. (Eds.). (1995). *Studying elites using qualitative methods.* Thousand Oaks, CA: Sage.

Hessler, R. M., Downing, J., Beltz, C., Pellicio, A., Powell, M., & Vale, W. (2003). Qualitative research on adolescent risk using email: A methodological assessment. *Qualitative Sociology, 26*(1), 111–124.

Hirsch, J., Higgins, J., Bentley, M. E., & Nathanson, C. A. (2002). Social constructions of sexuality: Marital infidelity and sexually transmitted disease—HIV
risk in a Mexican migrant community. *American Journal of Public Health, 92,*
1127–1237.

Hirsch, J. S., Meneses, S., Thompson, B., Negroni, M., Pelcastre, B., & Del Rio, C.
(2007). The inevitability of infidelity: Sexual reputation, social geographies,
and HIV marital risk in rural Mexico. *American Journal of Public Health, 97*(6):
986–996.

Hochschild, A., with Machung, A. (1989). *The second shift: Inside the two job marriage.*
New York: Avon.

Hohmann, A., & Shear, M. K. (2002). Community-based intervention research:
Coping with the "noise" of real life in study design. *American Journal of Psychiatry,*
159, 201–207.

Holland, J. (2007). Emotions and research. *International Journal of Social Research*
Methodology, 10, 195–209.

Hong, Y., Mitchell, S. G., Peterson , J. A., Latkin, C. A., Tobin, K., & Gann, D. (2005).
Ethnographic process evaluation: Piloting an HIV prevention program among
injection drug users. *International Journal of Qualitative Methods, 4*(1), Article 1.

Horowitz, C. R., Robinson, M., & Seifer, S. (2009). Community-based participatory
research from the margin to the mainstream: Are researchers prepared?
Circulation, 119(19), 2633–2642.

Hruschka, D. J., Schwartz, D., St. John, D. C., Picone-Decaro, E., Jenkins, R. A., &
Carey, J. W. (2004). Reliability in coding open-ended data: Lessons learned
from HIV behavioral research. *Field Methods, 16*(3), 307–331.

Humphries, L. (1970). *Tearoom trade: Impersonal sex in public places.* Chicago: Aldine.

Hunt, N., & McHale, S. (2007). A practical guide to the e-mail interview. *Qualitative*
Health Research, 17(10), 1415–1421.

Hyden, M., & Overlien, C. (2004). "Doing" narrative analysis. In D. K. Padgett (Ed.),
The qualitative research experience (pp. 250–268). Pacific Grove, CA: Thomson
Learning.

Illingworth, N. (2001). The Internet matters: Exploring the use of the Internet as a
research tool. *Sociological Research Online, 6*(2), U96–U112. Available at http://
www.socresonline.org.uk/6/2/illingworth.html

Inhorn, M. C., & Whittle, K. L. (2001). Feminism meets the "new" epidemiologies:
Toward an appraisal of antifeminist biases in epidemiological research on
women's health. *Social Science and Medicine, 53,* 553–567.

Inui, T. S., & Frankel, R. M. (1991). Evaluating the quality of qualitative research.
Journal of General Internal Medicine, 6, 485–487.

Irwin, L. G., & Johnson, J. (2005). Interviewing young children: Explicating our
practices and dilemmas. *Qualitative Health Research, 15*(6), 821–831.

Israel, B. A., Eng, E., Schulz, A. J., & Parker, E. A. (Eds.). (2005). *Methods in community-*
based participatory research for health. San Francisco: Jossey-Bass.

Iversen, R. R. (2009, March). "Getting out" in ethnography: A seldom-told story. *Qualitative Social Work, 8*(1), 9–26.

Iversen, R., & Armstrong, A. L. (2006). *Jobs aren't enough: Toward a new economic mobility for low-income families.* Philadelphia: Temple University Press.

Jacelon, C. S., & Imperio, K. (2005). Participant diaries as a source of data with older adults. *Qualitative Health Research, 15,* 991–997.

Janesick, V. J. (2000). The choreography of qualitative research designs: Minuets, improvisations, and crystallization. In N. K. Denzin & Y. S. Lincoln (Eds.), *Handbook of qualitative research* (2nd ed., pp. 379–400). Thousand Oaks, CA: Sage.

Johnson, P. J., & Onwuegbuzie, J. A. (2004). Mixed methods research: A research paradigm whose time has come. *Educational Researcher, 33*(7), 14–26.

Johnstone, P. L. (2004). Mixed methods, mixed methodology health services research in practice. *Qualitative Health Research, 14*(2), 259–271.

Jones, J. H. (1993). *Bad blood: The Tuskegee syphilis experiment.* New York: The Free Press.

Katz, J. (2006). Ethical escape routes for underground anthropologists. *American Ethnologist, 33*(4), 499–506.

Kelle, U., & Erzberger, C. (2004). Qualitative and quantitative methods: Not in opposition. In U. Flick, E. von Kardorff, & I. Steinke (Eds.), *A companion to qualitative research* (pp. 172–175). London: Sage.

Kelling, G. L., & Coles, C. M. (1996). *Fixing broken windows: Restoring social order and reducing crime in our communities.* New York: The Free Press.

Kerner, J. F., Yedidia, M., Padgett, D., Muth, B., Washington, K. S., Tefft, M., et al. (2003). Realizing the promise of breast cancer screening: Clinical follow-up after abnormal screening among Black women. *Preventive Medicine, 37,* 92–101.

Kidd, P. S., & Parshall, M. B. (2000). Getting the focus and the group: Enhancing analytical rigor in focus group research. *Qualitative Health Research, 10*(3), 293–308.

Kincheloe, J. L., & McLaren, P. (2000). Rethinking critical theory and qualitative research. In N. K. Denzin & Y. S. Lincoln (Eds.), *Handbook of qualitative research* (2nd ed., pp. 279–314). Thousand Oaks, CA: Sage.

Klinenberg, E. (2002). *Heat wave: A social autopsy of disaster in Chicago.* Chicago: University of Chicago Press.

Kotkin, S. (2002, September 7). A world war among professors: A clash between number crunchers and specialists in a single region. *New York Times,* pp. B9–B11.

Kozinets, R. V. (2010). *Netography: Doing ethnographic research online.* Thousand Oaks, CA: Sage.

Krieger, N. (2001). Theories for social epidemiology in the 21st century: An ecosocial perspective. *International Journal of Epidemiology, 30,* 668–677.

Krippendorf, K. (2004). *Content analysis: An introduction to its methodology* (2nd ed.). Thousand Oaks, CA: Sage.

Krueger, R. A. (1994). *Focus groups: A practical guide for applied research* (2nd ed.). Thousand Oaks, CA: Sage.

Kuhn, T. (1970). *The structure of scientific revolutions.* Chicago: University of Chicago Press.

Kurasaki, K. S. (2000). Intercoder reliability for validating conclusions drawn from open-ended interview data. *Field Methods, 12*(3), 179–194.

Kusenbach, M. (2003). Street phenomenology: The go-along as ethnographic research tool. *Ethnography, 4*(3), 455–485.

Labov, W., & Waletzky, J. (1967). Narrative analysis: Oral versions of personal experience. In J. Helm (Ed.), *Essays on the verbal and visual arts* (pp. 12–44). Seattle: University of Washington Press.

Ladson-Billings, G. (2000). Racialized discourses and ethnic epistemologies. In N. K. Denzin & Y. S. (Eds.), *Handbook of qualitative research* (2nd ed., pp. 258–278). Thousand Oaks, CA: Sage.

Laing, R. D. (1965). *The divided self: An existential study in sanity and madness.* London: Pelican Press.

Lakoff, G., & Johnson, M. (1980). *Metaphors we live by.* Chicago: University of Chicago Press.

LaPiere, R. T. (1934). Attitudes vs. actions. *Social Forces, 13,* 230–237.

LeCompte, M. D., & Schensul, J. J. (2010). *Analyzing and interpreting ethnographic data* (2nd ed.). Walnut Creek, CA: AltaMira Press.

Leung, M. W., Yen, I. H., & Minkler, M. (2004). Community-based participatory research: A promising approach for increasing epidemiology's relevance in the 21st century. *International Journal of Epidemiology, 33,* 1–8.

Levin, M., & Greenwood, D. (2001). Pragmatic action research and the struggle to transform universities into learning communities. In P. Reason & H. Bradbury (Eds.), *Handbook of action research* (pp. 103–113). London: Sage.

Levy, R. I., & Hollan, D. W. (2000). Person-centered interviewing and observation. In H. R. Bernard (Ed.), *Handbook of methods in cultural anthropology* (pp. 333–364). Walnut Creek, CA: AltaMira Press.

Lewin, K. (1946). Action research and minority problems. *Journal of Social Issues, 4,* 34–46.

Lewis, R. B. (2004). NVivo 2.0 and ATLAS.ti 5.0: A comparative review of two popular qualitative data analysis programs. *Field Methods, 16,* 439–464.

Liebow, E. (1967). *Talley's corner: A study of Negro street corner men.* Boston: Little, Brown.

Liebow, E. (1993). *Tell them who I am: The lives of homeless women.* New York: Penguin.

Lincoln, Y. S., & Guba, E. G. (1985). *Naturalistic inquiry.* Beverly Hills, CA: Sage.

Lincoln, Y. S., & Guba, E. G. (2000). Paradigmatic controversies, contradictions, and emerging confluences. In N. K. Denzin & Y. S. Lincoln (Eds.), *Handbook of qualitative research* (2nd ed., pp. 163–188). Thousand Oaks, CA: Sage.

Link, B. G., & Phelan, J. (1995). Social conditions as fundamental causes of disease. *Journal of Health and Social Behavior, 35,* 80–94.

Locke L., Spirduso, W., & Silverman, S. (1993). Preparation of proposals for qualitative research: Different assumptions. In L. Locke, W. Spirduso, & S. Silverman

(Eds.), *Proposals that work: A guide for planning dissertations and grant proposals* (3rd ed., pp. 96–118). Newbury Park, CA: Sage.

Lofland, J. (2002). Analytic ethnography. In A. M. Huberman & M. B. Miles (Eds.), *The qualitative researcher's companion* (pp. 137–170). Thousand Oaks, CA: Sage.

Lofland, J., & Lofland, L. (1995). *Analyzing social settings: A guide to qualitative observation and analysis* (3rd ed.). Belmont, CA: Wadsworth.

Luders, C. (2004). Field observation and ethnography. In U. Flick, E. von Kardorff, & I. Steinke (Eds.), *A companion to qualitative research* (pp. 222–230). London: Sage.

MacClean, L. M., Meyer, M., & Estable, A. (2004). Improving accuracy of transcripts in qualitative research. *Qualitative Health Research, 14*(1), 113–123.

MacGregor, T. E., Rodger, S., Cummings, A. L., & Leschied, A. W. (2006). The needs of foster parents: A qualitative study of motivation, support, and retention. *Qualitative Social Work, 5*(3), 351–368.

Mack, N., Woodsong, C., McQueen, K. M., Guest, G., & Namey, E. (2005). *Qualitative research methods: A data collector's field guide*. Research Triangle Park, NC: Family Health International. Available at http://www.fhi.org/en/rh/pubs/booksreports/qrm_datacoll.htm.

Madison, D. S. (2005). *Critical ethnography: Methods, ethics, and performance*. Thousand Oaks, CA: Sage.

Magnani, R., Sabin, K., Saidel, T., & Heckathorn, D. (2005). Review of sampling hard-to-reach and hidden populations for HIV surveillance. *AIDS, 19*(2), S67–S72.

Malinoswki, B. (1922). *Argonauts of the Western Pacific*. London: Routledge.

Malone, R. E., Yerger, V. E., McGruder, C., & Froelicher, E. (2006). "It's like Tuskegee in reverse": A case study of ethical tensions in institutional review board review of community-based participatory research. *American Journal of Public Health, 96*, 1914–1919.

Manderson, L., & Aaby, P. (1992). An epidemic in the field? Rapid assessment procedures and health research. *Social Science & Medicine, 35*, 839–850.

Manderson, L., Bennett, E., & Andajani-Sutjaho, S. (2006). The social dynamics of the interview: Age, class and gender. *Qualitative Health Research, 16*(10), 1317–1334.

Manderson, L., Kelaher, M., & Woelz-Stirling, N. (2001). Developing qualitative databases for multiple users *Qualitative Health Research, 11*(2), 149–160.

Manicas, P. T., & Secord, P. F. (1982). Implications for psychology of the new philosophy of science. *American Psychologist, 38*, 390–413.

Manwar, A., Johnson, B. D., & Dunlap, E. (1994). Qualitative data analysis with Hypertext: A case of New York City crack dealers. *Qualitative Sociology, 17*, 283–292.

Markham, A. N. (2005). The methods, politics, and ethics of representation in online ethnography. In N. K. Denzin & Y. S. Lincoln (Eds.), The SAGE *handbook of qualitative research* (3rd ed., pp. 793–820). Thousand Oaks, CA: Sage.

Marshall, C., & Rossman, G. B. (2006). *Designing qualitative research* (4th ed.). Thousand Oaks, CA: Sage.

Mathew, R. (2008). *Evolving traditions: South Asians and arranged marriages.* Youngstown, NY: Cambria Press.

Maxwell, J. (2002). Understanding and validity in qualitative research. In A. M. Huberman & M. B. Miles (Eds.), *The qualitative researcher's companion* (pp. 37–62). Thousand Oaks, CA: Sage.

Mayring, P. (2004). Qualitative content analysis. In U. Flick, E. von Kardorff, & I. Steinke (Eds.), *A companion to qualitative research* (pp. 266–270). London: Sage.

McCall, M. (2000). Performance ethnography: A brief history and some advice. In N. K. Denzin & Y. S. Lincoln (Eds.), *Handbook of qualitative research* (2nd ed., pp. 421–434). Thousand Oaks, CA: Sage.

McCoyd J. L., & Kerson, T. S. (2006). Conducting intensive interviews via email: A serendipitous comparative opportunity. *Qualitative Social Work, 5*(3), 389–406.

McCracken, G. (1988). *The long interview.* Newbury Park, CA: Sage.

McDonald, S. (2005). Studying actions in context: A qualitative shadowing method for organizational research. *Qualitative Research, 5*(4), 455–473.

McKibbon, K., & Gadd, C. (2004). A quantitative analysis of qualitative studies in clinical journals for the 2000 publishing year. *BMC Medical Informatics and Decision Making, 4*(1), 11–20.

McKinlay, J. (Ed.) (1986). *Issues in the political economy of health care.* London: Tavistock Publications.

Menand, L. (2001). *The metaphysical club: A story of ideas in America.* New York: Farrar, Straus & Giroux.

Merton, R. K., Fiske, M., & Kendall, P. (1956). *The focused interview.* Glencoe, IL: The Free Press.

Miles, M. B., & Huberman, A. M. (Eds.). (1994). *Qualitative data analysis: An expanded sourcebook* (2nd ed.). Thousand Oaks, CA: Sage.

Miller, D., & Slater, D. (2000). *The Internet: An ethnographic approach.* New York: Berg.

Miller, S. I., & Fredericks, M. (2006). Mixed-methods and evaluation research: trends and issues. *Qualitative Health Research, 16,* 567–579.

Mills, J., Bonner, A., & Francis, K. (2006). The development of constructivist grounded theory. *International Journal of Qualitative Methods, 5*(1), Article 3.

Minkler, M., & Wallerstein, N. (Eds.). (2003). *Community-based participatory research for health.* San Francisco: Jossey-Bass.

Mishler, E. (1986). *Research interviewing: Context and narrative.* Cambridge, MA: Harvard University Press.

Mitchell, W., & Irvine, A. (2008). I'm okay, you're okay? Reflections on the well-being and ethical requirements of researchers and research participants in conducting qualitative fieldwork interviews. *International Journal of Qualitative Methods, 7*(4), 31–44.

Morgan, D. L. (1997). *Focus groups as qualitative research.* Thousand Oaks, CA: Sage.

Morgan, D. L. (2007). Paradigms lost and pragmatism regained. *Journal of Mixed Methods Research, 1*(2), 48–76.

References 269

Morgan, D. L. (2010). Reconsidering the role of interaction in analyzing and reporting focus groups. *Qualitative Health Research, 20*(5), 717–722.

Morrow, S. (2005). Quality and trustworthiness in qualitative research in counseling psychology. *Journal of Counseling Psychology, 52*(2), 250–260.

Morrow, S. L., & Smith, M. L. (1995). Constructions of survival and coping by women who have survived childhood sexual abuse. *Journal of Counseling Psychology, 42*(1), 24–33.

Morse, J. M. (1991). Approaches to qualitative–quantitative methodological triangulation. *Nursing Research, 40,* 120–123.

Morse, J. M. (1994). Designing funded qualitative research. In N. K. Denzin & Y. S. Lincoln (Eds.), *Handbook of qualitative research* (pp. 220–235). Thousand Oaks, CA: Sage.

Morse, J. M. (1995). The significance of saturation. *Qualitative Health Research, 5,* 147–149.

Morse, J. M. (2004). Constructing qualitatively derived theory: Concept construction and concept typologies. *Qualitative Health Research, 14*(10), 1387–1395.

Morse, J. M. (2005). Evolving trends in qualitative research: Advances in mixed-method design. *Qualitative Health Research, 15*(5), 583–585.

Morse, J. M. (2006). The politics of evidence. *Qualitative Health Research, 16*(3), 395–404.

Morse, J. M. (2007a). Qualitative researchers don't count. *Qualitative Health Research, 17*(3), 287.

Morse, J. M. (2007b). Reasons for rejection, reasons for acceptance. *Qualitative Health Research, 17*(9), 1163–1164.

Morse, J. M. (2010). The clumsiness of measurement. *Qualitative Health Research, 20*(5), 871–872.

Munhall, P. L. (1994). *Qualitative research proposals and reports: A guide.* New York: National League for Nursing Press.

Moustakas, C. (1994). *Phenomenological research methods.* Thousand Oaks, CA: Sage.

Nader, L. (1969). Up the anthropologist: Perspectives gained from studying up. In D. Hymes (Ed.), *Reinventing anthropology* (pp. 284–311). New York: Random House.

Nastasi, B. K., & Hitchcock, J. (2009). Challenges of evaluating multilevel interventions. *American Journal of Community Psychology, 43*(3–4), 360–376.

Nelson, G., Ochocka, J., Griffin, K., & Lord, J. (1998). "Nothing about me, without me": Participatory action research with self-help/mutual aid organizations. *American Journal of Community Psychology, 26*(6), 881–913.

Newman, K., Fox, C., Roth, W., & Mehta, J. (2004). *Rampage: The social roots of school shootings.* New York: Basic Books.

Oakley, A. (1981). Interviewing women: A contradiction in terms. In H. Roberts (Ed.), *Doing feminist research* (pp. 30–61). London: Routledge & Kegan Paul.

Olesen, V. L. (2000). Feminisms and qualitative research at and into the millennium. In N. K. Denzin & Y. S. Lincoln (Eds.), *Handbook of qualitative research* (2nd ed., pp. 215–256). Thousand Oaks, CA: Sage.

Onken, S. J., Craig, C. M., Ridgway, P., Ralph, R. O., & Cook, J. A. (2004). *An analysis of the definitions and elements of recovery: A review of the literature.* Preconference paper prepared for the National Consensus Conference on Mental Health Recovery and Systems Transformation, Rockville, MD.

Padgett, D. K. (2004a). Mixed methods, serendipity and concatenation. In D. K. Padgett (Ed.), *The qualitative research experience* (pp. 269–281). Belmont, CA: Thomson.

Padgett, D. K. (Ed.). (2004b). *The qualitative research experience.* Belmont, CA: Thomson.

Padgett, D. K. (2004c). Spreading the word: Writing and disseminating qualitative research. In D. K. Padgett (Ed.), *The qualitative research experience* (pp. 285–296). Belmont, CA: Thomson.

Padgett, D. K. (2007). There's no place like (a) home: Ontological security in the third decade of the homelessness crisis. *Social Science & Medicine, 64,* 1925–1936.

Padgett, D. K. (2008). *Qualitative methods in social work research* (2nd ed.). Thousand Oaks, CA: Sage.

Padgett, D. K. (2009a). Qualitative and mixed methods in social work knowledge development. *Social Work, 54*(2), 101–105.

Padgett, D. K. (2009b). Qualitative methods in evaluation. In D. Royse, B. T. Thyer, D. K. Padgett, & T. K. Logan (Eds.), *Program evaluation* (5th ed., pp. 48–61). Pacific Grove, CA: Wadsworth.

Padgett, D. K., Conte, S., & Benjamin R. (2004). Peer debriefing and support groups. In D. K. Padgett (Ed.), *The qualitative research experience* (pp. 225–235). Belmont, CA: Thomson.

Padgett, D. K., Hawkins, R. L., Abrams, C., & Davis, A. (2006). In their own words: Trauma and substance abuse in the lives of formerly homeless women with serious mental illness. *American Journal of Orthopsychiatry, 76*(1), 461–467.

Padgett, D. K., Henwood, B., Abrams, C., & Davis, A. (2008). Engagement and retention in care among formerly homeless adults with serious mental illness: Voices from the margins. *Psychiatric Rehabilitation Journal, 31*(3), 226–233.

Padgett, D., Patrick, C., Burns, B. J., & Schlesinger, H. J. (1994). Ethnicity and use of outpatient mental health services in a national insured population. *American Journal of Public Health, 84,* 222–226.

Padgett, D. K., Stanhope, V., Henwood, B. F., & Stefancic, A. (2011, January 8). Substance use outcomes among homeless clients with serious mental illness: Comparing housing first with treatment first programs. *Community Mental Health Journal,* advance online publication, doi: 10.1007/s10597–009–9283–7.

Padgett, D. K., Yedidia, M., Kerner, J., & Mandelblatt, J. (2001). The emotional consequences of false positive mammography: African-American women's reactions in their own words. *Women and Health, 33,* 1–14.

Patton, M. Q. (2002). *Qualitative research and evaluation methods* (3rd ed.). Thousand Oaks, CA: Sage.

Perreault, M., Pawliuk, N., Veilleux, R., & Rousseau, M. (2006). Qualitative assessment of mental health service satisfaction: Strengths and limitations of a self-administered measure. *Community Mental Health Journal, 42*(3), 233–242.

Pinto, R. M. (2009). Community perspectives on factors that influence collaboration in public health research. *Health Education & Behavior, 36*(5), 930–947.

Pittaway, E., Bartolomei, L., & Hugman, R. (2010). Stop stealing our stories: The ethics of research with vulnerable groups. *Journal of Human Rights Practice, 2,* 229–251.

Polkinghorne, D. E. (1988). *Narrative knowing and the human sciences.* Albany: State University of New York Press.

Pope, C., & Mays, N. (1995). Reaching the parts other methods cannot reach: An introduction to qualitative methods in health and health services research. *British Medical Journal, 311,* 42–45.

Pope, C., Mays, N., & Popay, J. (2007). *Synthesizing quantitative and qualitative health research: A guide to methods.* London: Open University Press.

Punch, M. (1994). Politics and ethics in qualitative research. In N. K. Denzin & Y. S. Lincoln (Eds.), *Handbook of qualitative research* (pp. 83–97). Thousand Oaks, CA: Sage.

Putnam, G. (2000). *Bowling alone: The collapse and revival of American community.* New York: Simon & Schuster.

Rabinow, P., & Sullivan, W. M. (Eds.). (1979). *Interpretive social science: A reader.* Berkeley: University of California Press.

Ragin, C. C. (1987). *The comparative method. Moving beyond qualitative and quantitative strategies.* Berkeley: University of California Press.

Ragin, C. C., & Becker, H. S. (1992). *What is a case? Exploring the foundations of social inquiry.* Cambridge, UK: Cambridge University Press.

Rallis, S. F., & Rossman, G. B. (2003). Mixed methods in evaluation contexts: A pragmatic framework. In A. Tashakkori & C. Teddlie (Eds.), *Handbook of mixed methods in social and behavioral research* (pp. 491–512). Thousand Oaks, CA: Sage.

Rapkin, B. D., & Trickett, E. J. (2005). Comprehensive dynamic trial designs for behavioral prevention research with communities: Overcoming inadequacies of the randomized controlled trial paradigm. In E. J. Trickett & W. Pequegnat (Eds.), *Community intervention and AIDS* (pp. 249–277). New York: Oxford University Press

Raudenbush, S. W., & Bryk, A. S. (2002). *Hierarchical linear models: Applications and data analysis methods* (2nd ed.). Thousand Oaks, CA: Sage.

Reason, P., & Bradbury, H. (Eds.). (2007). *The SAGE handbook of action research* (2nd ed.). Thousand Oaks, CA: Sage.

Reinharz, R. (1992). *Feminist methods in social research.* New York: Oxford University Press.

Richardson, L. (2005). Writing: A method of inquiry. In N. K. Denzin & Y. S. Lincoln (Eds.), *The SAGE handbook of qualitative research* (3rd ed., pp. 959–978). Thousand Oaks, CA: Sage.

Ridgway, P. (2001). Re-storying psychiatric disability: Learning from first-person recovery narratives. *Psychiatric Rehabilitation Journal, 24*(4), 335–343.

Riessman, C. K. (1993). *Narrative analysis.* Newbury Park, CA: Sage.

Riessman, C. K., & Quinney, L. (2005). Narrative in social work: A critical review. *Qualitative Social Work, 4,* 391–412.

Rivera, R., & Borasky, D. (2009). *Research ethics training curriculum* (2nd ed.). Research Triangle Park, NC: Family Health International.

Rivera, R., Borasky, D., Rice, R., Carayon, F., & Wong, E. (2007). Informed consent: An international researcher's perspective. *American Journal of Public Health, 97*(1), 25–30.

Rolfe, G. (2006). Validity, trustworthiness and rigour: Quality and the idea of qualitative research. *Journal of Advanced Nursing, 53*(3), 304–310.

Rorty, R. (1998). *Truth and progress: Philosophical papers III.* Cambridge, UK: Cambridge University Press.

Ryan, G. W., & Bernard, H. R. (2000). Data management and analysis methods. In N. K. Denzin & Y. S. Lincoln (Eds.), *Handbook of qualitative research* (2nd ed., pp. 769–802). Thousand Oaks, CA: Sage.

Ryan, G. W., & Bernard, H. R. (2003). Techniques to identify themes. *Field Methods, 15*(1), 85–109.

Sacks, H., & Garfinkel, H. (1970). On formal structures of practical action. In J. C. McKinney & E. A. Tiryakian (Eds.), *Theoretical sociology* (pp. 338–366). New York: Appleton-Century-Crofts.

Saini, M., & Shlonsky, A. (2011). *Systematic syntheses of qualitative research.* New York: Oxford University Press.

Saldana, J. (2009). *The coding manual for qualitative researchers.* Thousand Oaks, CA: Sage.

Salmon, A. (2007). Walking the talk: How participatory interview methods can democratize research. *Qualitative Health Research, 17*(7), 982–994.

Sandelowski, M. (1993). Rigor, or rigor mortis: The problem of rigor in qualitative research revisited. *Advances in Nursing Science, 16,* 1–8.

Sandelowski, M. (2000). Combining qualitative and quantitative sampling, data collection, and analysis techniques in mixed methods studies. *Research in Nursing & Health, 23,* 246–255.

Sandelowski, M. (2002). Re-embodying qualitative inquiry. *Qualitative Health Research, 12*(1), 104–115.

Sandelowski, M., & Barroso, J. (2002). Reading qualitative studies. *International Journal of Qualitative Methods, 1*(1), Article 5.

Sandelowski, M., & Barroso, J. (2003). Classifying the findings in qualitative studies. *Qualitative Health Research, 13*(7), 905–923.

Sandelowski, M., & Jones, L. C. (1995). "Healing fictions": Stories of choosing in the aftermath of the detection of fetal anomalies. *Social Science and Medicine, 42,* 353–361.

Sanders, C. (2003). Application of Colaizzi's method: Interpretation of an auditable decision trail by a novice researcher. *Contemporary Nurse, 14,* 292–302.

Sands, R. G. (2004). Narrative analysis: A feminist approach. In D. K. Padgett (Ed.), *The qualitative research experience* (pp. 48–62). Belmont, CA: Thomson.

Sanjek, R. (1990). *Fieldnotes: The making of anthropology.* Albany: State University of New York Press.

Sarangi, S., & Candlin, C. (2003). Categorization and explanation of risk: A discourse analytical perspective. *Health, Risk & Society, 5*(2), 115–124.

Scheper-Hughes, N. (1996). Small wars and invisible genocides. *Social Science and Medicine, 43*(5), 889–900.

Schwandt, T. A., & Halpern, E. S. (1988). *Linking auditing and meta-evaluation: Enhancing quality in applied research.* Newbury Park, CA: Sage.

Scrimshaw, S. C., Carballo, M., Ramos, L., & Blair, B. A. (1991). The AIDS rapid anthropological assessment procedures: A tool for health education planning and evaluation. *Health Education Quarterly, 18*(1), 111–123.

Scrimshaw, S. C., & Gleason, G. R. (1992). *Rapid assessment procedures: Qualitative methodologies for planning and evaluation of health-related programs.* Boston: International Nutrition Foundation for Developing Countries (INFDC).

Seidman, I. (2006). *Interviewing as qualitative research.* New York: Teachers College Press.

Shibusawa, T., & Lukens, E. (2004). Analyzing qualitative data in a cross-language context: A collaborative model. In D. K. Padgett (Ed.), *The qualitative research experience* (pp. 175–186). Belmont, CA: Thomson.

Shibusawa, T., & Padgett, D. K. (2009). Out of sync: A life course perspective on aging among formerly homeless adults with serious mental illness. *Journal of Aging Studies, 23,* 188–196.

Shiellerup, P. (2008). Stop making sense: The trials and tribulations of qualitative data analysis. *Area, 40,* 163–171.

Silverman, D. (2006). *Interpreting qualitative data* (3rd ed.). Thousand Oaks, CA: Sage.

Singer, M., & Clair, S. (2003). Syndemics and public health: Reconceptualizing disease in bio-social context. *Medical Anthropology Quarterly, 17*(4), 423–441.

Slevin, E., & Sines, D. (2000). Enhancing the truthfulness, consistency and transferability of a qualitative study: Utilising a manifold of approaches. *Nurse Researcher, 7*(2), 79–89.

Snow, D. A., & Anderson, L. (1991). Researching the homeless: The characteristic features and virtues of the case study. In J. R. Feagin, A. M. Orum, & G. Sjoberg (Eds.), *A case for the case study* (pp. 148–173). Chapel Hill: University of North Carolina Press.

Spradley, J. P. (1979). *The ethnographic interview.* New York: Holt, Rinehart & Winston.

Stake, R. E. (1995). *The art of case study research.* Thousand Oaks, CA: Sage.

Stake, R. E. (2005). *Multiple case study analysis.* New York: Guilford Press.

Stange, K. C., Miller, W. L., Crabtree, B. F., O'Connor, P. J., & Zyzanski, S. J. (1994). Integrating qualitative and quantitative research methods. *Family Medicine, 21,* 448–451.

Stein, A. (2010). Sex, truths, and audiotape: Anonymity and the ethics of exposure in public ethnography. *Journal of Contemporary Ethnography, 39*(5), 554–568.

Steinmetz, A. M. (1991). Doing. In M. Ely, M. Anzul, T. Friedman, D. Garner, & A. M. Steinmetz (Eds.), *Doing qualitative research: Circles within circles* (pp. 41–68). London: Falmer Press.

Strauss, A., & Corbin, J. (1990). *Basics of qualitative research: Grounded theory procedures and techniques.* Newbury Park, CA: Sage.

Strauss, A., & Corbin, J. (1994). Grounded theory methodology: An overview. In N. K. Denzin & Y. S. Lincoln (Eds.), *Handbook of qualitative research* (pp. 273–285). Thousand Oaks, CA: Sage.

Stringer, E. T. (2007). *Action research: A handbook for practitioners* (3rd ed.). Thousand Oaks, CA: Sage.

Szreter, S., & Woolcock, M. (2004). Health by association? Social capital, social theory, and the political economy of public health. *International Journal of Epidemiology, 33,* 1–18.

Tannen, D. (1990). *You just don't understand: Women and men in conversation.* New York: William Morrow.

Tannen, D. (2006). *You're wearing that? Understanding mothers and daughters in conversation.* New York: Ballantine Books.

Tashakkori, A., & Creswell, J. W. (2007). The new era of mixed methods. *Journal of Mixed Methods Research, 1*(1), 3–7.

Tashakkori, A., & Teddlie, C. (Eds.). (2010). *SAGE handbook of mixed methods in social and behavioral research* (2nd ed.). Thousand Oaks, CA: Sage.

Taylor, J. (2007). Assisting or compromising intervention? The concept of culture in biomedical and social research on HIV/AIDS. *Social Science & Medicine, 64*(4), 965–975.

Taylor, S. J. (1987). Observing abuse: Professional ethics and personal morality in field research. *Qualitative Sociology, 10,* 288–302.

Taylor, S. J., & Bogdan, R. (1984). *Introduction to qualitative research: The search for meanings* (2nd ed.). New York: Wiley.

Tedlock, B. (2000). Ethnographic and ethnographic representation. In N. K. Denzin & Y. S. Lincoln (Eds.), *Handbook of qualitative research* (2nd ed., pp. 455–486). Thousand Oaks, CA: Sage.

Ten Have, P. (1999). *Doing conversation analysis.* London: Sage.

Teram, E., Schachter, C. L., & Stalker, C. A. (2005). The case for integrating grounded theory with participatory action research: Empowering clients to inform professional practice. *Qualitative Health Research, 15*(8), 1129–1140.

Tesch, R. (1990). *Qualitative research: Analysis types and software tools.* London: Falmer Press.

Thorne, S. (1998). Ethical and representational issues in qualitative secondary analysis. *Qualitative Health Research, 8*(4), 547–555.

Thorne, S., Jensen, L., Kearny, M. H., Noblit, G., & Sandelowski, M. (2004). Qualitative metasynthesis: Reflections on methodological orientation and ideological agenda. *Qualitative Health Research, 14*(10), 1342–1365.

Tjora, A. H. (2006). Writing small discoveries: An exploration of fresh observers' observations. *Qualitative Research, 6*(4), 429–451.

Travers, K. D. (1997). Reducing inequities through participatory research and community empowerment. *Health Education & Behavior, 24*(3), 344–356.

Trickett, E. J. (2009). Multilevel community-based culturally situated interventions and community impact: An ecological perspective. *American Journal of Community Psychology, 43*(3–4), 257–266.

Twinn, S. (1997). An exploratory study examining the influence of translation on the validity and reliability of qualitative data in nursing research. *Journal of Advanced Nursing, 26*, 418–423.

Uehara, E. (2001). Understanding the dynamics of illness and help-seeking: Event structure analysis and a Cambodian American narrative of "spirit invasion." *Social Science and Medicine, 52*, 519–536.

Ulin, P. R., Robinson, E. T., & Tolley, E. E. (2005). *Qualitative methods in public health: A field guide for applied research.* San Francisco: Jossey-Bass.

Ungar, M. (2006). "Too ambitious": What happens when funders misunderstand the strength of qualitative research design. *Qualitative Social Work, 5*(2), 261–277.

Van den Berg, Harry (2005). Reanalyzing qualitative interviews from different angles: The risk of decontextualization and other problems of sharing qualitative data [48 paragraphs]. *Forum Qualitative Sozialforschung / Forum: Qualitative Social Research, 6*(1), Art. 30. Available at http://www.qualitative-research.net/index.php/fqs/article/view/499.

Van Maanen, J. (1988). *Tales of the field: On writing ethnography.* Chicago: University of Chicago Press.

Van Manen, M. (Ed.). (2002). *Writing in the dark: Phenomenological studies in interpretive inquiry.* London, Ont., Canada: Althouse.

Van Manen, M. (2006). Writing qualitatively, or the demands of writing. *Qualitative Health Research, 16*, 713–722.

Victora, C. G., Habicht, J., & Bryce, J. (2004). Evidence-based public health: Moving beyond randomized trials. *American Journal of Public Health, 94*(3), 400–405.

Waldrop, D. (2004). Ethical issues in qualitative research with high-risk populations. In D. K. Padgett (Ed.), *The qualitative research experience* (pp. 236–249). Belmont, CA: Thomson.

Walker, D., & Myrick, F. (2006). Grounded theory: An exploration of process and procedures. *Qualitative Health Research, 16*(4), 547–559.

Wang, C. C., Morrel-Samuels, S., Hutchinson, P., Bell, L., & Pestronk, R. M. (2004). Flint photovoice: Community building among youths, adults, and policymakers. *American Journal of Public Health, 94*(6), 911–914.

Wang, C. C., & Redwood-Jones, Y. A. (2001). Photovoice ethics: Perspectives from Flint photovoice. *Health Education and Behavior, 28*(5), 560–572.

Waters, E., & Doyle, J. (2002). Evidence-based public health practice: Improving the quality and quantity of evidence. *Journal of Public Health Medicine, 24*(3), 227–229.

Weiss, R. S. (1994). *Learning from strangers: The art and method of qualitative interview studies.* New York: The Free Press.

Weitzman, E., & Miles, M. (1995). *Computer programs for qualitative data analysis: A software sourcebook.* Thousand Oaks, CA: Sage.

West, C. (1989). *The American evasion of philosophy: A genealogy of pragmatism.* Madison: University of Wisconsin Press.

White, M., & Epston, D. (1990). *Narrative means to therapeutic ends.* New York: Norton.

Whittemore, R., Chase, S. K., & Mandle, C. (2001). Validity in qualitative research. *Qualitative Health Research, 11*(4), 522–527.

Williams, C. C., & Collins, A. A. (2002). The social construction of disability in schizophrenia. *Qualitative Health Research, 12*(3), 297–309.

Willis, K., Daly, J., Kealy, M., Small, R., Koutroulis, G., Green, J., et al. (2007). The essential role of social theory in qualitative public health research. *Australian and New Zealand Journal of Public Health, 31*(5), 438–443.

Willis, K., Green, J., Daly, J., Williamson, L., & Bandyopadhyay, M. (2009). Perils and possibilities: Achieving best evidence from focus groups in public health research. *Australian and New Zealand Journal of Public Health, 33*(2), 131–136.

Wilson, H. S., & Hutchison, S. (1991). Triangulation of qualitative methods: Heideggerian hermeneutics and grounded theory. *Qualitative Health Research, 1*, 263–276.

Wimpenny, P., & Gass, J. (2000). Interviewing in phenomenology and grounded theory: Is there a difference? *Journal of Advanced Nursing, 31*(6), 1485–1492.

Wolcott, H. F. (2009). *Writing up qualitative research* (3rd ed.). Thousand Oaks, CA: Sage.

World Health Organization. (2000). *Operational guidelines for ethics committees that review biomedical research.* Geneva, Switzerland: Author.

Yin, R. K. (Ed.). (2004). *The case study anthology.* Thousand Oaks, CA: Sage.

Yin, R. K. (2008). *Case study research: Design and methods* (4th ed.). Thousand Oaks, CA: Sage.

Index

Note: Page numbers in *italics* refer to figures or boxes of information.

About the Author

Deborah K. Padgett, a professor at New York University's Silver School of Social Work, received her doctorate in anthropology and completed postdoctoral training programs in public health and psychiatric epidemiology at Columbia University and Duke University. A mental health services researcher, Dr. Padgett has published extensively on the health/ mental health needs and service use of underserved ethnic groups, women, and the homeless. In addition to previous National Institutes of Health (NIH) grants, she is currently Principal Investigator of an all-qualitative R01 grant from the National Institute of Mental Health (NIMH) to study recovery and the service delivery system for homeless adults with co-occurring mental and substance use disorders in New York City. In addition to this text, Dr. Padgett is the editor of a reader in qualitative methods, *The Qualitative Research Experience* (2004), and *The Handbook of Ethnicity, Aging, and Mental Health* (1995), and she is coauthor of *Program Evaluation* (fifth edition, 2009). Her expertise in qualitative methods has led to contributions to several NIH Training Institutes and grant reviews. Dr. Padgett has also been an active mentor of other researchers and has served on numerous journal editorial boards. Currently, she is Interim Director of New York University's Masters in Global Public Health program where she teaches courses in socio-behavioral health and qualitative/ field methods.

SAGE Research Methods Online
The essential tool for researchers

**Sign up now at
www.sagepub.com/srmo
for more information.**

An expert research tool

- An **expertly designed taxonomy** with more than 1,400 unique terms for social and behavioral science research methods

- **Visual and hierarchical search tools** to help you discover material and link to related methods

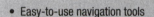

- Easy-to-use navigation tools
- Content organized by complexity
- Tools for citing, printing, and downloading content with ease
- Regularly updated content and features

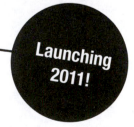

A wealth of essential content

- The most comprehensive picture of quantitative, qualitative, and mixed methods available today

- More than **100,000 pages of SAGE book and reference material** on research methods as well as editorially selected material from SAGE journals

- More than **600 books** available in their entirety online

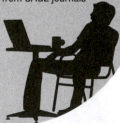

Launching 2011!

⑤SAGE research methods online